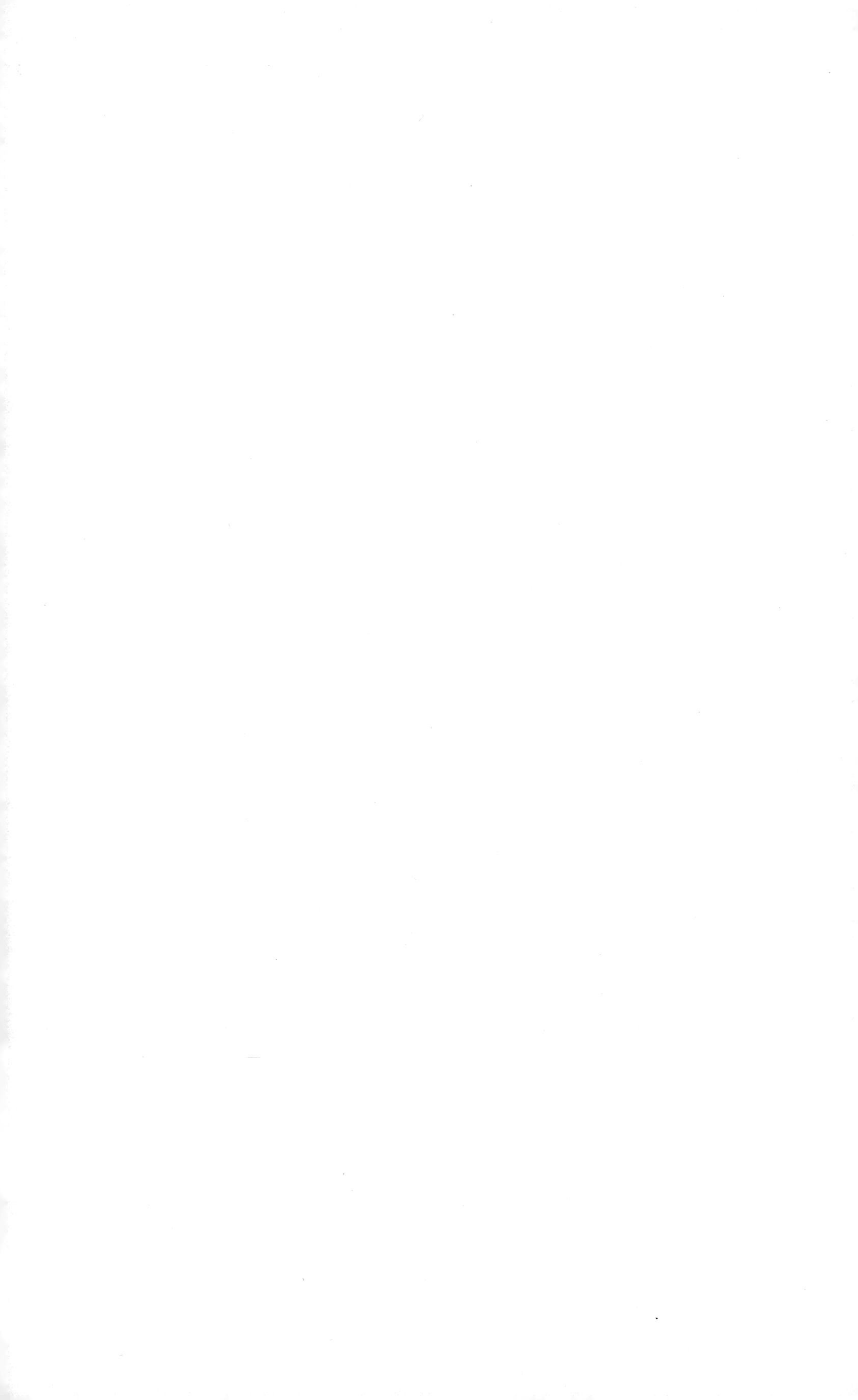

Twenty-Two Years

Twenty-Two Years

Causes and Consequences of Mental Retardation

Stephen A. Richardson
and
Helene Koller

Harvard University Press
Cambridge, Massachusetts
London, England
1996

Printed in the United States of America

Library of Congress Cataloging-in-Publication Data

Richardson, Stephen A.
Twenty-two years : causes and consequences of mental retardation / Stephen A. Richardson and Helene Koller.
p. cm.
Includes bibliographical references and index.
ISBN 0-674-21297-5
1. Mental retardation—Etiology. I. Koller, Helene. II. Title.
[DNLM: 1. Mental retardation—Complications.]
RC570.2.R53 1996
616.85′88071—dc20 96-28834

To the young people and their parents
who took part in this study

Contents

Preface

This book reports on a follow-up study of young people with mental retardation (MR). The period covered is the first twenty-two years of life. Our purposes are to examine the histories and personal characteristics of these young people, to obtain a comprehensive perspective on how the various aspects of their lives are related to one another, to determine the prevalence and distribution of MR, and to seek clues to the causes of MR. The study is unique in that it is based on a representative population of young people with MR of all degrees of severity and examines their lives in childhood, as well as when they were young adults, from biological and psychosocial perspectives. The book builds on a series of journal publications and book chapters based on this research, each of which was written for a particular audience and dealt with a specific topic.

We believe the study is of interest and relevance to the diverse group of people who know and are concerned about individuals with MR: parents and other relatives, educators, social workers, physicians, psychologists, and other professionals responsible for the care of children and adults with mental retardation. All get to know some aspects of some people with MR, even if only for limited periods of time. We also believe that the study has broad relevance for those interested in child development, epidemiology, and life course studies.

We recognize that readers will approach this book with particular interests related to their own background and training, and we have tried to organize it so that the information they are looking for is easily available. We have also tried to limit our use of technical terms and to define those we do use.

Background

An important earlier study, described more fully in Chapter 1, provided the opportunity and the impetus for the present research. To focus and frame the present study, we selected concepts and theory that would guide us in selecting and analyzing the data (see Chapter 2). In Chapter 3 we review the methods and results used in previous follow-up studies in order to gain from previous investigative experience. Other reviews of research are included in later chapters as they relate to specific topics. These reviews enabled us to compare the present with past results. Chapter 4 describes the design and methods of the present study.

Epidemiology

The young people in our study constituted a total representative population of all those with MR at a defined time and place. They were identified using epidemiological methods, which enabled us to determine their prevalence in the community and how it varied by age, gender, severity of MR, and whether children with MR were over- or underrepresented in certain kinds of families within the community. Our results add to the body of knowledge that may be used to estimate the prevalence of MR in other communities. The prevalence and distribution of MR are described in Chapter 5. Because one of the purposes of epidemiology is to provide clues to cause, in Chapter 6 we examine a number of factors with etiological implications.

Individual Characteristics

In addition to the degree of severity of MR in the individuals in the study, we were interested in whether their IQ's were generally stable during childhood or whether there was appreciable change. We were also interested to learn about other forms of disability and the frequency with which these occurred either singly or in combination. Some disabilities were present for only part of the time up to age twenty-two, so we examined these disabilities in terms of stability and change at different ages. We also wanted to know about their appearance and how these young people felt about themselves at age twenty-two, so we developed measures of appearance and self-esteem. We wanted to know how these measures compared with those of peers who did not have MR and any related factors in their histories. Chapters 7 through 13 deal with individual characteristics.

Histories

We focused first on the family, because it plays such an important role in the socialization of children. Another important influence on the lives of the young people in the study was the educational system, especially the forms of special education that were provided for children with MR. Children who were considered unable to benefit from special education received alternative MR services.

We wanted to know how many young adults did and did not continue to receive MR services after school-leaving age. We especially wanted to know what happened to those young adults who did not receive adult services, and we examined their histories in some detail. An important question concerned the quality of their lives—whether the young adults who were not in MR services led lives similar to or different from those of their peers who did not have MR. We examined this question as it related to job histories and activities outside of work hours, and in terms of friendships and marriage. Chapter 14 deals with families, Chapter 15 examines the mental retardation service histories of the young people, and Chapters 16 and 17 deal with job histories and activities outside of working hours.

Because we followed children into adulthood, we were able to determine how well we could predict adult adjustment from personal characteristics and childhood histories and also examine relationships between different facets of their lives. These analyses are the subject of Chapter 18. When we had completed the four major sections of the book, we examined the extent to which the study results are still relevant today.

During the years of the study, we were privileged to gain the confidence and cooperation of the individuals who formed the study population and of their parents. We are deeply grateful to them for telling us so much about themselves and have been vigilant in safeguarding the data we collected as well as those we obtained from other research and administrative sources. The largely quantitative presentation of the results protects the anonymity of individuals. When we felt it necessary to illustrate some of the findings with brief case histories, we were always careful to change any identifying information while maintaining the features that illustrated the particular point we were making.

The study described in this book would not have been possible without the help of a large number of people and organizations over a period of more than thirty-five years.

The ideas for the study were initiated at the Association for the Aid of Crippled Children (AACC), an endowed foundation in New York City with a mandate "to further understanding of the causes and consequences of handicapping conditions, especially in children." In the 1950s, as the Assistant Director of the AACC, Stephen A. Richardson worked closely with three outstanding consultants—Herbert Birch, M.D., Ph.D., Ernest Gruenberg, M.D., Ph.D., and Chester Swinyard, M.D., Ph.D.—whose joint expertise included psychology, pediatrics, psychiatry, epidemiology, statistics, anatomy, genetics, and physical medicine. The AACC board, under the direction of Leonard Mayo, encouraged him, along with the three consultants, to develop and recommend policy objectives. To further understanding of mental retardation (MR), the group agreed that an epidemiological study of a total population of children with MR would be an important form of research for the foundation to support, and the board concurred.

The reasons Aberdeen was chosen as the study site are described in Chapter 1 and in *Mental Subnormality in the Community* (Birch et al. 1970). The final planning of that study was carried out by Herbert Birch and Stephen Richardson in collaboration with Sir Dugald Baird, Professor of Obstetrics at the University of Aberdeen and Honorary Director of the Obstetric Medicine Research Unit of the British Medical Research Council, and Raymond Illsley, Ph.D., a sociologist in the research unit. Many members of the faculty at the university served as consultants to the study. The preface to *Mental Subnormality in the Community* gratefully acknowledges more than fifty individuals and organizations whose contributions provided the basis for the follow-up study.

We recognized that obtaining funds for a follow-up study would be a major problem. Funding agencies are aware that longitudinal studies are a high-risk venture and may take many years; it is safer to fund research more limited in scope and duration. Our study also entailed many inherent problems, such as tracing the individuals to be studied over a long time span, maintaining continuity in the staffing of the research team, and meeting high research costs. Before funding a follow-up study, an agency may reasonably ask for evidence from pilot studies that the individuals to be studied can be traced and, when located, will cooperate with investigators. Because of the imaginative vision of the AACC, later renamed the Foundation for Child Development (FCD), we were able to carry out a pilot study of a sample of children with histories of mental retardation who were now young adults. When Richardson moved to Albert Einstein College of Medicine, the FCD set aside a block of funds for him to draw upon as he saw fit, as long as the research complied with the FCD mandate. Some of these funds were used for the pilot study, and they also made it possible to retain a core staff, because salaries could be underwritten and maintained during the intervals when other funding dried up.

The study design called for a five-year period of data gathering. We realized that it would be unlikely that any funding agency would commit funds beyond five years without clear evidence that the data had been successfully collected. For this reason, our initial request was for five years of funding. In 1972, the William T. Grant Foundation and the National Institute of Child Health and Human Development (HD07970, 07907) provided the funds needed for data gathering, and we are indebted to them for taking the risk.

After the initial funding, obtaining support in order to analyze and write up the results proved difficult. Some agencies were unwilling to fund such work when they had not been involved in gathering data. We were unable to find any agency that would make a general grant to fund the range of analyses we envisaged, but we eventually succeeded in obtaining funds by packaging the overall analysis into smaller, specific pieces, and tailoring our requests to the policies and interests of particular agencies. We are grateful for the financial support we received from the following agencies: the Charitable Trust of Mrs. Abby Mauze, the G. Harold and Leila Mathers Charitable Foundation, the National Institute of Child Health and Human Development, the William T. Grant Foundation, the Foundation for Child Development, the Bowen and Jan McCoy Foundation, and the Thomas and Mary Alice O'Malley Foundation. In the United Kingdom, we obtained funding from the Scottish Home and Health Department and from the Social Science Research Council.

We owe a special debt to Raymond Illsley. As Professor of Sociology and Honorary Director of a new Medical Sociology Research Unit of the Medical Research Council, he made the administrative resources of his research unit available to us. He also helped organize the pilot study, with Janice Boath as the interviewer. The results were sufficiently encouraging for us to undertake a full follow-up study.

The collection of the research data involved many organizations and individuals, and we are deeply grateful to all of them. The University of Aberdeen agreed to administer the research funds and provided the policies under which the research team members were employed. In his Medical Sociology Research Unit, Professor Illsley generously provided us with office space and administrative support. Several of his colleagues gave us valuable help and consultation. We particularly want to thank Gordon Horobin, Barbara Thompson, and Mike Samphier.

The first person hired for the staff at Aberdeen was Janice McLaren. She assisted in developing the interview and observation schedules, in selecting and training the team of interviewers, and acted as deputy for Richardson when he was in New York. Later, she participated in the data coding and in the early phases of analysis. We want to thank her for her dedication to the research and her organizational and leadership skills, and for the key role she played on the research team.

Eight interviewers participated in the study: Diana Summers, Rosemary Dawson, Joan Seal, Brenda Parsons, Barbara Stroud, Barbara Fraser, Margaret Mannings, and Betta Adams. In addition to taking on the largest number of interviews in Aberdeen, Diana Summers also interviewed those living in other parts of the United Kingdom. The interviewers' work was taxing intellectually, emotionally, and physically, and we want to thank all of them for the competent and cheerful way in which they carried out a difficult task.

Irene Easton and Harry Johnston checked interviews, organized the incoming data, and collected further data from documentary sources. Edna Sassella did the typing. The coding of the data, a major task requiring accuracy and painstaking attention to detail, was carried out with the assistance of Sharon Wardell, Helen Oliver, Martha Campbell, and Harry Johnston. The staff maintained a high standard of work and we are most grateful to them.

The work of the entire research team was marked by friendly and congenial relationships, which made being with them a privilege and a great pleasure.

Many human services professionals in Aberdeen were extremely helpful and gave generously of their time to facilitate our research.

These include Dr. James Clark, Director of Education in the city; Ian McKinnon, and his successor, Winifred Ferrier, who were in charge of special education; Dr. Harold Ross, Director of the MR residential institution for children; and Dr. Allen Cook, who directed the MR residence for adults. Dr. Allen Clark, the senior psychologist at the adult institution, was a valuable consultant to our work. The staff at the Senior Occupation Centers facilitated some of the interviewing.

In the Aberdeen Department of Social Work, we were aided by Douglas Grant and Charles Lingham. Ross Henderson of the Youth Employment Service assisted us in learning about employment in Aberdeen.

At the University of Aberdeen, we received assistance from Dr. Ross Mitchell, Professor of the Department of Child Health, and his successor, Dr. Alex Campbell. Dr. John Nisbet, Professor of Education, consulted with us on intelligence tests and the educational system in Scotland. Dr. Malcolm Miller, Professor of Mental Health, consulted with us on the mental health services available in Aberdeen. Later in the project, Dr. George Innes of the Department of Community Medicine gave us office space.

The authors' home base was the Social Ecology Research Unit, directed by Richardson, in the Kennedy Center for Research in Mental Retardation and Human Development at Albert Einstein College of Medicine. Mindy Katz was a key and valued colleague who brought her expertise in biostatistics and data management to the research and worked with us in the unit during the analysis of data. Other staff members, Ann Barnecott and Lisa Harrington, were excellent secretaries and also helped with the coding of data. Two research fellows at Einstein—Dr. Keith Goulden and Dr. Boris Rubenstein—made important contributions to our research. Dr. Goulden, a pediatric neurologist, helped gather medical research data in Aberdeen, assisted in developing categories from the data, and collaborated in writing the chapters on etiology and epilepsy. Dr. Rubenstein, a pediatric psychiatrist, helped us to develop the classification of behavior disturbance and to code the relevant research data, and also participated in the analysis.

We also received help from graduate students and volunteers. Ronda Facchini developed the self-esteem measure and used it as the basis for her doctoral thesis, while Joanne Kaufmann, Amy Weintraub, Michael Stowe, and Jeffrey Schlesinger helped at various stages of the analysis. We thank them all. Lucinda Ash, ever patient, did the typing and retyping, including the tables, and her accuracy and care proved crucial in developing the final manuscript.

We were fortunate to be working at the Kennedy Center, where scientists from widely diverse backgrounds were engaged in research related to mental retardation. They generously advised us on the wide range of topics in this book. We especially want to thank Drs. Dominick Purpura, Herbert Vaughan, and John Kessler, the directors of the Kennedy Center during our tenure there; Dr. Harold Nitowski, who consulted with us on genetics; Dr. Isabelle Rapin, who consulted on autism; Dr. Arnold Birenbaum, who consulted on medical sociology; and Dr. Herbert Cohen, who consulted on pediatrics and developmental disabilities.

We also received assistance from other colleagues at Einstein who were not based at the Kennedy Center: Dr. Schlomo Shinnar, a pediatric Neurologist, consulted with us on epilepsy and collaborated on Chapter 9. Drs. Jay Selman and Daniel Adler helped to code some of the epilepsy data. Dr. Sylvia W. Smoller consulted with us in epidemiology and statistics, and Dr. Ruth Macklin on ethics.

The authors were members of the Department of Pediatrics at Einstein and were given encouragement and administrative support by Drs. Henry Barrett, Chester Edelman, and Michael Cohen, who each in turn served as department chair. We are grateful to them for their support.

We developed close ties with the Department of Epidemiology in the School of Public Health at Columbia University, and want to thank Drs. Mervyn Susser, Zena Stein, and William Hauser for valuable consultation.

Through correspondence and occasional meetings, we were helped by Professors Jack Tizard at the University of London, Alan and Anne Clarke at the University of Hull, and Bengt and Gudrun Hagberg at the University of Gothenborg.

At Harvard University Press we received valuable help from Angela von der Lippe, who encouraged us over the years; Linda Howe, whose judicious editing has improved the text; and Elizabeth Gretz, who shepherded the manuscript through production.

For permission to reprint brief portions of earlier publications related to this research, we are grateful to Waverly International, for the use of material from Birch et al. (1970); and to the American

Association on Mental Retardation and the *American Journal on Mental Retardation,* for the use of material from Koller et al. (1983); Koller, Richardson, and Katz (1992); Richardson, Katz, and Koller (1986b, 1993); and Richardson, Koller, and Katz (1985a, c; 1988).

Our deepest debt of gratitude is to the hundreds of young adults in the study and to their parents. They gave us hours of their time, and even more important, they gave us their trust by sharing with us their histories, their concerns, and their feelings.

Part I

Background

1

A Research Opportunity

The present study had its origins in the research reported in *Mental Subnormality in the Community—A Clinical and Epidemiological Study* (Birch et al. 1970). The purposes of the earlier study were to

1. determine the prevalence of mental subnormality in a defined age range
2. describe the mentally subnormal children thus identified in terms of the degree of severity of their mental defect and the presence or absence of associated clinically demonstrable signs of central nervous system damage and psychiatric disorder
3. examine the degree to which mental subnormality and its association, or lack of association, with clinically demonstrable neurologic and psychiatric disorder was distributed in various social segments of the community
4. examine the association of obstetric and perinatal antecedents with mental subnormality and its associated neurologic features
5. examine the interrelations of social, familial, and health conditions in mental subnormality and its subvariants
6. identify interactions between the biological and social factors associated with mental subnormality (p. 5)

The community in which the research was carried out necessarily had to meet two important criteria. First, investigators had to be able to identify and study every child in the community who met a commonly accepted definition of mental retardation.[1] Second, they needed access to records of the obstetrical and perinatal events related to the birth of children who did and did not have mental retardation. These records, in addition, had to have been collected at the time they occurred in a standardized form suitable for research purposes. During the search for an appropriate community, the investigators came across the research publications of Sir Dugald Baird, professor of obstetrics at the University of Aberdeen. He was studying the epidemiology of complications of pregnancy and delivery and had obtained standardized records of every pregnancy and delivery in the city. Fortunately, he agreed to cooperate in the study.

The researchers then examined the mental retardation services in the city itself and found that their records, policies, and practices met the first need of identifying a population of children with mental retardation. The Education and Health Authorities also agreed to cooperate with the study. Aberdeen seemed to be an outstanding community for our research purposes.

Obstetrical and Perinatal Events

One difficulty in studying the events that may contribute to the etiology of mental retardation is that, especially in its milder forms, mental retardation may remain unidentified until the school years. Two study designs were considered.

> One approach is to start with the population of children who are identified as mentally subnormal and move back in time to determine the antecedent events associated with mental subnormality by comparing this population of children with those in the same birth years who are not mentally subnormal. Alternatively, one can begin with certain complications of pregnancy, delivery, or early childhood which, on the basis of previous research and theory, are believed to contribute to the development

1. "Mental retardation" is one of a series of synonyms that have been used over time to refer to this condition. As each term has developed negative connotations and come to seem derogatory and stigmatizing, it has been replaced by another. Examples include "mental deficiency," "mental handicap," "mental subnormality," and "intellectual disabilities." The term currently in use the United Kingdom is "learning disability," but we will follow contemporary usage in the United States and use "mental retardation."

> of mental subnormality, and follow up those children at presumed risk to determine whether mental subnormality occurs more often in association with a given complication than in its absence. The first approach begins with children who are mentally subnormal and leads back in a search for causal factors. The alternative design begins with "factors" believed to contribute to the causes of mental subnormality and traces their consequence forward in time. (Birch et al. 1970, pp. 20–21)

Given the purposes of the study, researchers chose the first approach, starting with the population of children with mental retardation as the point of reference. This strategy was made possible because of the existence in Aberdeen of a unique body of maternity and health records, which had been systematically collected over many years.

> After the end of World War II, a number of events took place that made it possible to develop a system of record collection and storage to provide information on the social background, pregnancies, and deliveries of the total population of Aberdeen. Moreover, the establishment of the National Health Service in 1947 resulted in a considerable degree of unification of obstetric care. Many services were transferred to the Maternity Hospital, which shortly came to provide antenatal and maternity services for more than 85 per cent of all pregnancies in the city. Maternity care for domiciliary births was provided by the National Health Service. Cooperation of midwives, general practitioners, and obstetricians was good and all records of these non-hospital births are transferred to the Maternity Hospital on special forms matched to the Maternity Hospital records. Since 1948, all maternity records have been coded and placed on punchcards, thus making them readily available for statistical analysis. Opportunities for the acquisition, organization, and processing of maternity data for the total population of the city were improved in 1948 by the establishment of a Medical Research Council Research Team, especially devoted to obstetric research. This team, which, from its inception included an epidemiologist and a statistician, was augmented in 1951 to include a full-time research sociologist. Consequently, since that date, the obstetric records have included sociologic information, much of which is obtained routinely on all cases, and some of which was collected for given

samples on an ad hoc basis in connection with special studies. (pp. 19–20)

Defining Mental Retardation

A primary requirement of the study was a method of identifying every child who met a given definition of mental retardation (MR). For the purposes of the study, children were defined as MR if they had been identified as such by the local educational and health authorities and placed in a special school or other facility for children with MR. A small number of children with MR, however, did not attend these facilities and were kept at home by joint agreement of the parents and local authorities.

This "administrative" definition depends on the identification process used by the local authorities. In 1962, when the children were studied, segregation of children with MR in special schools was an accepted practice, as was the widespread use of IQ testing for educational assessment. Children with severe MR were identified, in most cases prior to school entry age, by the local health authorities in conjunction with an educational psychologist. Children with mild MR were identified predominantly during the early school years. Unless it was apparent that a child had mental retardation prior to school age, all children entered school in regular classes, where teachers were asked to notify the education authorities if, in their judgment, any child appeared to have mental retardation.

A second method of identification used the group intelligence tests given to every child in the city at ages 7, 9, and 11. Any child scoring below 75 on these tests was referred for individual psychometric assessment. Because teachers varied in their willingness to refer pupils as possibly having MR, the test scores on the group intelligence tests served as a backup identification method. After all referred children had been given a psychometric assessment by the school psychologist, the report of the assessment was sent to the school medical officer, who evaluated the child's whole situation by relating the psychological findings to the child's current health, past history, and all other examination results. As part of the general evaluation procedure, the school medical officer asked the head of the child's school to submit information on his or her school achievement along with any additional information, such as behavior or patterns of play, that was felt to be pertinent to the evaluation. The head of the school could also make a recommendation as to the child's proper school placement.

> The evaluation and general recommendation together with the psychologic test information and other pertinent data are recorded on a standard form for statutory reasons. The completed form, the supporting material from the psychologist, the contributions of the headmaster, and the recommendation of the School Medical Officer are then sent to the Director of Education, who reviews the entire case. He discusses the situation with the child's parents and makes his own recommendation to the Education Committee.
>
> If the Education Committee approves the recommendation, the Director of Education is free to implement it. The Director of Education is required to communicate with the parents in writing, stating his recommendation and its basis and pointing out to them their right to appeal against the decision—first to the educational authorities in Aberdeen and then, if they wish, to the Secretary of State for Scotland. When an appeal is made to the Secretary, his representatives review the entire dossier and make an independent judgment. Their decision is then sent in writing to the parents, with a copy to the educational authorities.
>
> In addition to the statutory procedure described above, there is a system of voluntary referral. If they wish, parents may send their child to a special school . . . on a trial basis, in order to determine whether such an arrangement is in his best interests. If the parents are not satisfied with their child's progress in the special school, they can insist that he be returned to a regular school. If, on the other hand, they feel that placement in the special school is appropriate, voluntary referral can be made statutory . . .
>
> The criteria used in the Aberdeen screening and evaluation of children reflect the view that no single measure is adequate and that identification must be based upon an overall evaluation of the child—that is, his intellectual, physical, and social functioning as well as his school performance. Clearly, the classification of a child as mentally subnormal may be influenced by the nature of the special educational facilities that are available. If the special physical and personnel resources are overtaxed or inferior in quality, teachers, physicians, and parents may be reluctant to identify and categorize a child as mentally subnormal. Such a classification would be pointless if no special facilities

> existed for the child or even harmful if it placed the child in overcrowded or inadequate settings. This bias in classification is unlikely to occur in Aberdeen because of the generous provision of physical facilities for the mentally subnormal and because of the quality of the teaching staff.
>
> The general attitude in Aberdeen toward the teaching of handicapped children has been that it calls for a high level of skill and experience on the part of teachers. Only those who are experienced and successful in teaching normal school children and who express a strong interest in handicapped children are selected for special training. The teacher remains on salary and all training costs are borne by the educational authorities. Those teachers who successfully complete the special training earn a higher salary than do teachers in the regular schools. (Birch et al. 1970, pp. 18–19)

A small number of children attended private schools. The city director of education was responsible for overseeing both municipal and private schools, and both types used the same administrative procedures for classifying children as MR.

Although few children who were classified as MR were placed in residential facilities, it was possible that some of these children might have been placed in residences outside the geographic boundaries of Aberdeen and thus might be omitted from the authorities' records. When this possibility was looked into, however, it was ascertained that local authorities were responsible for keeping in touch with all children placed in residences outside of Aberdeen whose parents resided in the city. It was only after an investigation into the procedures used in classifying children as mentally retarded that the study definition of mental retardation was adopted.

Some epidemiological studies of mental retardation use only a psychometric definition: all children with an IQ below a given cutoff point, often IQ 70, are defined as having MR. The availability of intelligence test scores for every child in Aberdeen made it possible to identify all children who were not administratively defined as having MR but had IQ's below a given IQ cutoff point.

Selection of the Study Population

Approximately 3,000 children entered school each year in Aberdeen. In the initial study, it was estimated that approximately 100 children with mental retardation were needed, and that this number would be obtained from three birth cohorts of children. The study population was defined as all children born in the years 1952 through 1954 who were resident in Aberdeen in 1962. Their ages thus ranged from 8 to 10 years. It was felt that by that time, all children with mental retardation would have been identified.

To determine the prevalence of mental retardation, it was necessary to know the total number of children in Aberdeen born during the years 1952–1954 and still resident in the city in 1962, and to determine the number of children per 1,000 with mental retardation. Information on the total number of children in the three birth cohorts was obtained from the annual census of all Aberdeen children carried out by the education authorities.

Assessments of Children's Impairments

Group intelligence tests given to every school child at ages 7 and 9 provided IQ data. As part of their assessment, all children suspected of having mental retardation were then tested by a school psychologist prior to classification as mentally retarded. The children thus classified were subsequently given IQ tests at intervals throughout their childhood.

For research purposes, it was felt important to obtain independent evaluations of the children. Using the Wechsler Intelligence Scale for Children (WISC), an American team of psychologists evaluated the total population of children born from 1952 to 1954 who had been administratively defined as MR. They concluded that all had been correctly classified. The research team also obtained a psychiatric and, independently, a neurologic assessment of every child identified as mentally retarded through individual examinations. In the psychiatric assessment, a history of the child's behavior was also obtained by interviewing the child's teacher and/or caretaker. In the neurological assessment, a standardized clinical neurological schedule was used.

Children's Health Histories

The city Department of Health administered a Health Visitor Service. By statute, specially trained nurses were required to make home visits to every child in Aberdeen several times a year from his or her birth to school entry. Systematic records of these visits were maintained, and these revealed the dates at which children attained developmental landmarks, evidence of significant illnesses, and indications of the adequacy of child care. Once children had entered the school system, the school medical officer was responsible for evaluating their health and maintaining records for all children throughout their school career. Hospital records were also available for those children who had been hospitalized.

Access to Health and Other Human Services

Poor access to services may contribute to the causes of mental retardation. In many places, access may be limited either because services are lacking or because an individual is unable to pay for them. At the time of the study, health and other services in Aberdeen were of good quality and, because they had been nationalized, were available to all without individual payment.

Minority Groups and Recent Foreign Immigrants

In communities where there are minority groups who experience discrimination, these social conditions may increase the likelihood that children may be identified as having mental retardation. Children who are recent immigrants to different cultures, where the language is different, may also be at greater risk of being identified as having mental retardation. The extent to which these conditions exist in a community complicates, and possibly confounds, the study of mental retardation. At the time of the study, there were no distinct minority groups in Aberdeen and few immigrants from other countries.

The knowledge about Aberdeen gained during the course of the first study was invaluable when we considered following the children into adulthood. A number of factors influenced the decision to do so. Widespread geographic dispersion can render follow-up studies hazardous because many individuals become lost to follow-up, but separate research on migration patterns in Aberdeen showed that the city's population was stable. We were also fortunate that the various local authorities worked in close cooperation with each other, that the city had a tradition of research, and that university faculty and those responsible for services had a working relationship of mutual trust and respect. Since we had already been involved in research in the city, we were known throughout the community. As a result, research workers, local authorities, and those providing services generously offered their cooperation and assistance in the follow-up study.

2

Issues and Concepts

Etiology

One focus of the research in Birch et al. (1970) was the etiology of mental retardation (MR). At that time, researchers were greatly interested in determining whether complications of pregnancy and delivery were important etiological factors in MR. They were also interested in psychosocial adversity experienced by infants and children during their upbringing as an etiological factor. Birch et al. showed that obstetrical complications did not deserve the importance attached to them in the thinking of the time. The etiological role of specific genetic conditions, such as Down syndrome, was already recognized. Strong associations were found, however, between aspects of potential psychosocial adversity and mild MR for children whose neurologic assessment showed no evidence of central nervous system damage. For other children with MR, the authors concluded that

> a proportion of cases of subnormality can be attributed to central nervous system damage, which, in turn, can be attributed to severe obstetrical complications . . . obstetric complications might well have been the significant etiologic factor in one-quarter of the neurologically-damaged group, although it is possible that an adverse post-natal environment also made a contribution in at least some cases (p. 165) . . . It is clear that in [upper social classes], approximately one-half of the general population,

> the causes of very severe damage must be found elsewhere than in clinically recognizable obstetric factors in the majority of cases. (Birch et al. 1970, p. 153)

We saw a further opportunity for etiologic research in the data we collected during the follow-up. Research carried out after the Birch et al. study had shown the contributions of intergenerational genetic and chromosomal disorders, such as the fragile-X syndrome, to MR. We felt that the additional data warranted further etiological investigation.

The Histories of Young People with Mental Retardation

Previous research has made it clear that the histories of young people with severe MR (IQ <50) will, in general, be very different from those with mild MR (IQ ≥50). Those with severe MR continue to need supervision and support from their families and service providers as adults, and will not become completely self-supporting and independent. Especially when they have additional disabilities, those with severe MR place a heavy burden on the people responsible for their daily care. We took these issues into account in planning the kind of information we would gather for histories of individuals with MR.

The histories of young adults with mild MR are more diverse. Some information comes from studies of those known to adult mental retardation service agencies because they needed services. Those who were in institutions have histories that were heavily dependent on the policies and practices of those institutions; with the shift away from institutional placement to a wide variety of community services, however, the particular form of service again became a major influence.

Less is known about the adults with mild MR who disappear from mental retardation services when they leave special education. It is often difficult to find them unless they were known to researchers as children or could be traced from school records. In a review of the epidemiology of mental retardation, Gruenberg (1964) considered the young people with MR who received no further mental retardation services after school-leaving age. As he pointed out, in a number of epidemiological studies the prevalence of mental retardation after age 14 was only half as high as that at age 14. Because all, or almost all, of those with severe MR receive adult MR services, considerably more than half of those with mild MR disappear from MR services when they reach school-leaving age. These findings pose critical questions not only for understanding the nature of mental retardation but for public policy decision making. Gruenberg suggested, for example, that

> For this drop in prevalence to occur, a large group of people regarded as retarded at fourteen must improve in their functioning to the point where people no longer regard them as retarded and also must succeed in escaping their history of earlier unsatisfactory performance . . . Either these individuals are continuing to be extremely handicapped in later life and are unknown because the services they need are unavailable to them (in which case society is failing to do its duty toward them and ought to learn how to find and help them), or they have stopped being retarded in any real sense at all and do not need any special protection, help or services, in which case one had better change one's concept of what "real" mental retardation "really" is . . . [The phenomenon] cries out for investigation. (p. 274)

For purposes of emphasis, Gruenberg suggested two widely different alternatives. What is more likely is that adult adjustment will be distributed across the range of these two extremes. Thirteen years later, a group of consultants to the National Institute of Child Health and Human Development repeated and expanded Gruenberg's plea for follow-up studies of children with mental retardation: "Life span studies of the mentally retarded must be undertaken because little is known about the life pattern of the retarded, particularly those who are not institutionalized" (Ad Hoc Consultants 1977, p. 5).

If there is wide variability in the adult histories of those who disappear from MR services after leaving school, it would be important to account for the fact that some individuals do better than others. One may examine this issue by determining how varied the histories are, what aspects of childhood predict specific adult outcomes, and what adult characteristics are associated with how these individuals function in daily activities. The ideas presented thus far suggest several questions for a study following children with mental retardation into adulthood:

1. What are their histories after leaving school?
2. Why do some young adults do better than others?

3. Among those who disappear from services, how similar or different are they in their postschool histories from peers who came from a similar social milieu but did not have mental retardation?

It was also important to examine the histories of the young people before and during their school years; in this way we hoped to determine whether factors that could aid in the etiological analysis were present and to consider the question of why some young adults do better than others.

Selecting Salient Factors in the Histories

Once we had determined the general purposes of the study, the next step was to select salient factors in the life histories. One frequently used research method is to base variable selection on a theory, or theoretical construct, from which hypotheses are derived. We could find no single theory that was sufficiently comprehensive to encompass our interests. In addition, over the twenty-year span covered by the study—from its initial planning to the final analysis and writing up of results—there have been advances in theory, knowledge, and analytical techniques. Wherever appropriate, we have attempted to take advantage of these advances. As an overall framework, we used three general concepts proposed by Homans (1950, 1961)—activities, interactions, and sentiments—and selected aspects of the histories relevant to each concept.

Activities

Educational and vocational activities. The general expectation is that children in Aberdeen between the ages of 5 and 15 will be engaged in educational activities five days a week and that those beyond the age of compulsory education will engage in a vocational activity—or continue for some time in further education or training in preparation for a vocation. The role of housewife, which may or may not include the bearing and rearing of children, is considered a vocation. For those who cannot meet these expectations, certain day and residential care facilities are provided.

Evening, weekend, and holiday activities. During waking hours, in the time not devoted to educational or vocational activities, a wide variety of other activities are customary and socially acceptable, including the pursuit of personal and social interests, hobbies, and sports. These activities may be solitary or shared, and may take place inside or outside an organizational or institutional context. There are also some activities that are proscribed, either formally or informally, by the society as a whole or within particular subcultures.

Interactions

It is generally expected that children and young adults will be involved in a variety of interpersonal relationships and will develop functional and affectional ties with others. The following general categories of interactions were explored in the life histories but within the context of friendships; affectional ties; sources of help, guidance, or support; and recalled interactions in which an individual was bullied, teased, made fun of, or taken advantage of. These are

1. interactions related to or stemming from educational or vocational activities and evening, weekend, and holiday activities
2. affiliations to informal groups, clubs, organizations, churches
3. relationships stemming from residence in some institution, such as a facility for people with MR or psychiatric illness, or living and working on a ship or in prison
4. family relationships, subdivided among one's family of orientation (both primary and extended) and through marriage to one's family of procreation and spouse's family of orientation (both primary and extended)
5. interactions (other than with family) related to place of residence, such as with neighbors
6. interactions initiated in connection with obtaining or providing goods and services, or through casual encounters in public places

Sentiments

Sentiments include personal reaction to, judgments toward, and evaluation of activities and interactions; self-evaluation; and fulfilled and unfulfilled goals and aspirations. In the interviews, a distinction was maintained between obtaining an account of activities and interactions (evidence), and the personal evaluation of the particular event (inference and subjective reaction), such as how the young people felt about their families, schooling, and job histories.

We were also guided by socialization theory (Clausen 1968). Very little was known about the life course of young people with MR up to young adulthood and how they make the critical developmental changes expected of young people in our society. These changes include

1. a shift in social relations away from their families of origin toward other social relationships, especially with nonfamily peers
2. a shift from schooling to an adult occupational career
3. a shift from economic dependence on parents toward economic independence
4. a shift toward the assumption of responsibility for personal planning and actions, and management of personal affairs, including being a law-abiding citizen.
5. the development of heterosexual relationships, marriage, and parenting
6. shifts in the use of leisure time

Later, we found a valuable articulation and clarification of how our conceptual thinking was developing in Bronfenbrenner's (1979) *Ecology of Human Development*:

> The ecology of human development involves the scientific study of the progressive accommodation between an active, growing organism and the changing properties of the immediate settings in which the developing person lives, as this process is affected by relations between these settings, and by the larger contexts in which the settings are embedded. (p. 21)

The definition of human ecology is similar in some of its elements to the host-environment interaction, a concept that has been widely used in epidemiology. It differs, however, in its emphasis on the organism's longitudinal accumulation of experience as a child, and later as an adult, and in the distinction between environmental factors that directly and indirectly interact with the child or adult. This conceptual perspective may be seen in schematic form as a time clock that moves from conception and birth to childhood and adulthood (see Figure 2.1). The face of the clock is divided into concentric circles: the inner circle represents the characteristics of the individual, which include, for example, the person's gender and any impairments he or she may have; the outer circle represents the social and physical environment the individual experiences over time, either directly or indirectly. Direct experiences, for example, would be provided by parents and friends, or by the kind of housing in which the child lives, while indirect experiences would include the kind of job the child's parents hold, and the conditions of the job market.

The present study focuses in general on the intermediate concentric circle, which represents the outcome of the interaction between the individual and his or her environment (for example, job history,

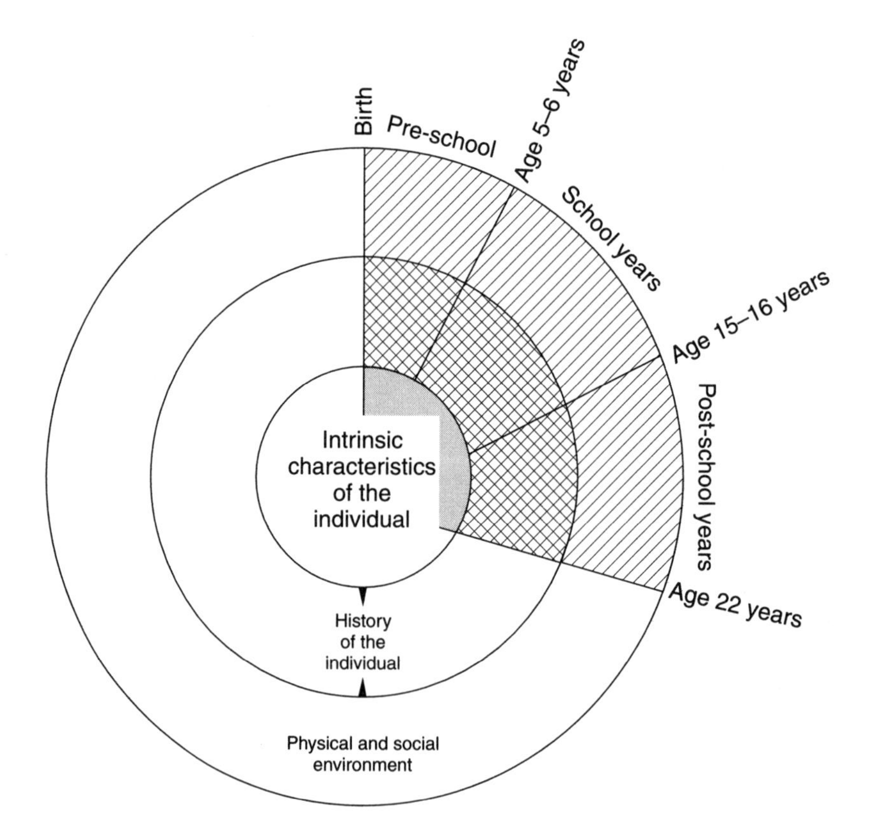

Figure 2.1 Schematic representation of the life course from birth to age 22, showing how the intrinsic characteristics of the individual and the physical and social environments influence the history of the individual. Reprinted from Richardson et al. 1990.

friendships, and leisure-time activities). It is also possible to look at some of the particular characteristics of the family environment, such as the health histories of the parents. Because for most young people there is a major shift in roles after school-leaving age, we examine the school years separately from the postschool years.

Epidemiologic Concepts

The study of Birch et al. (see Chapter 1), which was based on epidemiologic concepts, provided an unusually solid foundation for the present study, including, most significantly, a well-defined population representative of all the children living in a geographic area at a given time and with given birth years. (See Chapter 5 for a full description of the epidemiologic concepts used in the present study.) The selection procedures encompassed children with mental retardation of all levels of severity, from mild to profound. Information about all the children in these birth cohorts living in Aberdeen enabled us to select appropriate nonretarded peers for comparative purposes, determine the prevalence of mental retardation and its subtypes in the city, and examine how the children with mental retardation were distributed by social class. Because intelligence test scores were available for every child in the city, we could determine the number of children who were not administratively classified as having mental retardation and thus remained in regular classes, but who on psychometric grounds alone could be considered to have mental retardation.

Future chapters dealing with specific aspects of these young people's lives will include additional theory and concepts relevant to the topic. In addition to using concepts and theory as a basis for our data collection, we also benefited from a pilot follow-up study using intensive life history interviews obtained from the young people themselves and their parents. Careful examination of these data consolidated our theoretical thinking and revealed other topics of inquiry that, given our theoretical orientation, we had previously overlooked.

3

Previous Research

The research studies we reviewed were selected because of their relevance to the present study. First we will consider studies that followed children with mild MR who disappeared from MR services after school-leaving age, and then studies of children with MR who did not disappear from these services. Although many studies were carried out between 1910 and the late 1960s, research following up on children from special schools came to a virtual halt in the ensuing years.

Children with Mental Retardation Who Disappeared from MR Services

The question of what happens to children with mental retardation after they leave special classes or schools has been asked since early in this century. Ramer (1946) reviewed fourteen such studies carried out in the Scandinavian countries and Germany between 1911 and 1930. These investigations were generally conducted by teachers of special classes who were concerned about what happened to their pupils after they left school. What they generally asked was whether their former pupils would be able to support themselves, a question based on the then current definitions of mental retardation. In England and the United States, the definitions were similar to that used in Scandinavia: a person was considered mentally retarded if he was not qualified to look after himself and attend to his own affairs (Ramer, 1946, p. 12). Reviewing the results of the studies, however, Ramer found a number of problems:

1. Lack of uniformity in the standards used in deciding to place children in special classes.
2. Differences in the prevailing conditions of the time and in the social environment.
3. Variation in authors' interpretation of their results.
4. The omission of a comparable group of nonretarded peers for comparison.
5. Data of questionable validity.
6. Collection of data only from the pupils most easily traced, and thus unrepresentative.

None of the follow-up studies reviewed by Ramer included nonretarded persons for comparative purposes, and this was also true for many studies carried out later in the United Kingdom.

For special attention we selected four follow-up studies, all of which included nonretarded adults for comparison and were carried out when study subjects were in their twenties, the ages of the subjects of the present study. These studies were also among the more carefully designed and executed of those available. We also reviewed an additional study that did not meet these requirements because it demonstrated important conceptual and methodological differences from the other studies.

The potential range of questions that might be asked about the life course of a child with mental retardation up to young adulthood is enormous. When investigators consider what salient issues they wish to study, they are influenced by some mix of contemporary and traditional values, beliefs, and information about mental retardation. We will refer to this mix as the "conventional wisdom." Conventional wisdom also influences how researchers interpret their results. Before reviewing the follow-up studies, we will describe the conventional wisdom about mental retardation at the time of the earlier studies and the changes that had occurred by the time of the later studies.

Conventional Wisdom about Mental Retardation

Two influential studies, one by Richard L. Dugdale (1877) and one by Henry Goddard (1912), emphasized the heritability of traits. Among the families he studied, Dugdale found "a preponderance of pauperism, harlotry, illegitimate children, syphilis, deformed youngsters and a higher crime rate among the offspring." Goddard, who obtained similar results, concluded, "Feeble-mindedness is hereditary and transmitted as surely as any other character. We cannot successfully cope with those conditions until we recognize feeble-mindedness and its hereditary nature, recognize it early, and take care of it" (quoted in Scheerenberger 1983, p. 150).

Early in the twentieth century, Sir Francis Galton developed an eugenics theory that widely influenced thinking about mental retardation. Eugenics was conceived of as a scientific way of improving human stock by giving "the more suitable strains of blood a better chance of prevailing speedily over the less suitable." This thinking was encouraged by the successful results of selective breeding by farmers and horticulturists. Galton believed that "the processes of evolution are in constant and spontaneous activity, some towards the bad, some towards the good. Our part is to watch for opportunities to intervene by checking the former and giving free play to the latter" (Kevles 1984a, p. 51).

Motivated by eugenics theory, Charles Davenport, in the United States, carried out extensive studies on family pedigrees to investigate the genetic makeup of individuals. Whenever he found a high incidence of a given character in a family pedigree, he concluded that the trait must be heritable. Under the umbrella of "heritable" traits he included alcoholism, feeble-mindedness, prostitution and loose sexual morals, criminality, a general nervous weakness, and pauperism, which was considered to result from "relative inefficiency," a term used to indicate mental inferiority (Kevles 1984a, p. 101).

Walter Fernald, an influential figure in the field of mental retardation, expressed the conventional wisdom that had grown out of these studies and the eugenics movement.

> The past few years have witnessed a striking awareness in professional and popular conscience of the widespread prevalence of feeble-mindedness and its influence as a source of wretchedness to the patient himself and to his family, and as a causative factor in the production of crime, prostitution, pauperism, illegitimacy, intemperance and other complex social diseases . . . The feeble-minded are a parasitic, predatory class, never capable of self-support or of managing their own affairs. The great majority ultimately become public charges in some form. They cause unutterable sorrow at home and are a menace and a danger to a community (quoted in Scheerenberger 1983, p. 157).

By 1918, however, Fernald had tempered this harsh view: "there are both bad feeble-minded and good feeble-minded, and . . . not all of the feeble-minded are criminalist and socialists and immoral and antisocial . . . We know that a lot of the feeble-minded are generous, faithful and pure-minded" (p. 158).

Fernald's more pessimistic assessment of the unchangeable, lifelong nature of mental retardation still existed in the early 1940s. When, in the 1930s and 1940s, the Nazis embraced the ideas of eugenics and selective breeding of human stock, however, their actions were so shocking they set off a strong negative reaction to eugenics. With the swing away from genetics as the primary factor in mental retardation, other biological and psychosocial factors were increasingly emphasized. The effects of psychosocial adversity were considered less immutable and more subject to change if later experiences provided a more favorable psychosocial environment. From an early, highly pessimistic prognosis for children with mild MR, there was a shift toward greater optimism. Yet, as we will see, the conventional wisdom about mental retardation continued to influence research workers and reviewers of research.[1]

Four Follow-up Studies Using Nonretarded Comparisons

The first of the four studies (Fairbanks, 1933) was carried out in the early 1930s in Baltimore, Maryland, and reported in *The Subnormal Child—Seventeen Years After.* The 166 children in the study had been selected as subnormal and in need of special training from the general community school population of 1,281 children. These 166 children had been the subjects of a 1914 study, which had divided them into three groups. The first group, those with the most pronounced mental defects, included 22 children with an average IQ of 61, approximately 2 percent of the school population. All but 5 of this group attended ungraded classes in the public school, and most of them had a family history of feeblemindedness, alcoholism, or immorality. Many had special physical handicaps, showed delinquency traits, and were unable to read or write or do an errand. The children in this group were expected to have no prospect of becoming self-supporting adults and considered liable to be among "the ranks of the vagrants, the alcoholics, the prostitutes, and the delinquents." The second group was made up of 78 children with somewhat less

1. The language and terminology used by the earlier researchers have been left unchanged.

glaring limitations, and thus more widely distributed throughout the grades. Their average IQ was 72. It was anticipated that later in life they would be found "drifting along at the lowest social level." The third, least handicapped group of 66 children also had an average IQ of 72, but it was felt that they had "greater possibility of economic efficiency," although, as potential delinquents, the somewhat higher level of their intelligence also increased the possibility that they might be "detrimental to society" (Fairbanks, 1933, pp. 179–180). The influence of the conventional wisdom on these assumptions is apparent. At the time of Fairbanks's follow-up, the study population was in their twenties.

The initial design of the study included no nonretarded peers for comparative purposes. At the completion of the follow-up of the subnormal children, however, "a question was raised as to the scientific value or significance of the study without a control group to show wherein our conclusions were valid or might perhaps be too optimistic an interpretation of the facts" (p. 195). In response to this criticism, Fairbanks added a "normal" control group made up of children from the same school with IQ's of 90 and above who were not considered to have MR.

Fairbanks obtained the following results when the children were followed-up as young adults. Compared with peers who did not have MR,

1. more of the subnormal group had married and had more children and more divorces.
2. promiscuity, prostitution, and illegitimacy are somewhat more frequent in the subnormal group.
3. there is a larger percentage of affiliations with social agencies among the subnormals. About 10 per cent are receiving financial aid, while none of the control group requires this assistance. The subnormal individual also needs more personal guidance.
4. although almost as many of the subnormal as of the normal group are self-supporting, living conditions in the normal group as a whole are much more comfortable.
5. about two-thirds of the subnormals earn their living as laborers, while an equal proportion of the normals have superior jobs.
6. a larger percentage in the subnormal group have juvenile court records, while the incidence of police court records is about

the same for the two groups. There is more alcoholism, but less social drinking among the subnormals.

7. the fact that more of the normal group have migrated to other parts of the city, that they have superior jobs, and that they show more variety in their interests and recreations is apparently due to a difference in personality make-up in the two groups, as well as to somewhat greater economic ease in the control group. (Fairbanks, 1933, p. 204)

In her comments on the results, Fairbanks points to the discrepancy between the school authorities' expectations that the children would "be shiftless, alcoholic, of low wage-earning capacity, and dependent on charitable organizations for support," and her findings, which revealed a somewhat remarkable degree of stability when these children were followed up later. She speculates on the factors that may have accounted for the results:

> The atmosphere of respectability and community pride in a small town-like setting, the effects of these contacts in the early years with teachers who were not convictionless, but aggressively determined not to lose an opportunity to inculcate good old-fashioned morality, embodying principles of decency and respect for individual personality and clearmindedness . . . In scrutinizing the results that seventeen years of life experience have brought about in this group of . . . subnormal boys and girls, we must not allow ourselves to overemphasize the discrepancy between the rather sober prophecies made years ago concerning their future, and the actual outcome. Those predictions were based upon what experience has shown does befall the defective child exposed to the merciless struggle for livelihood and happiness in the world at large . . . Here, in an unusually constructive environment located in the industrial center of a city, we find a group of children with particularly poor endowment and unfavorable outlook developing into men and women who show a somewhat remarkable degree of stability. The lessons they have taught should sink deeply into our group consciousness and reawaken a faith in the responsiveness of human nature. (pp. 207–208)

In Fairbanks's comments we see clearly the influence of the conventional wisdom.

The second study, carried out by Baller (1936), followed up children who had been in special classes in the public schools of Lincoln, Nebraska, in 1916. They had IQ's below 70 and had been classified as having MR by the school psychologist. At follow-up, they ranged in age from 21 to 34 years. As nonretarded comparisons, Baller selected children in the same public school system with IQ's between 100 and 120 and matched them with children who had been classified as MR on gender, age, and nationality, but not the social class of their parents. Baller's summary and conclusions reported the following results. At follow-up, in contrast to their comparisons, those with MR more often came from families in which the wage earner was employed in unskilled and often irregular labor, there was more antisocial behavior in the family, they had more siblings,the family was more often broken up by divorce, more of those with MR had died, fewer of the males had married, women married earlier and had more children, they exhibited more antisocial conduct, and fewer had relatively permanent employment. They moved more often within the neighborhood but less often away from the neighborhood (pp. 232–234).

In reviewing Fairbanks's study, Baller wrote, "This report gives a particularly bright picture of the prospects of successful adjustment on the part of individuals, who, in school, may be classified as mentally subnormal" (p. 189). Baller also made a broader evaluation of this study and the other, previous studies he reviewed: "A final appraisal of the findings would warrant the judgment that many persons of subnormal intelligence can be successfully adjusted to community life although local conditions of many kinds will alter the results and such factors as previous training and present supervision are important." This statement suggests that individuals with MR play a passive rather than an active role in their later adjustment. With the knowledge of the results of Fairbanks's study and his own, Baller appears to have been influenced far less by the pessimistic conventional wisdom.

The third study was carried out by Ramer (1946) in Stockholm, Sweden, at the end of World War II and reported in *The Prognosis of Mentally Retarded Children.* In his review of earlier European follow-up studies of "backward" children as adults, Ramer pointed out a number problems that made it difficult to interpret the studies, (see p. 3.2). In his own study, he attempted to overcome these problems.

His aim was to find out how many children in special classes had failed in life. One purpose of his study was to be " . . . an aid to the assessment of the eugenic measure that should be taken to produce a healthy generation" (p. 69). In the next sentence, however, he also shows his concern for environmental factors: "Moreover, such investigations are a necessary part of child psychiatry and other mental hygiene which is intended to improve the living conditions of the mentally retarded individual and his adjustment to society" (p. 69).

Ramer focused attention in his follow-up study on marriage, means of support, need for public relief, insanity, criminality, vagrancy, and inebriation. Study subjects were selected from among those who had attended special classes "intended for mentally retarded children unable to follow the instruction given in normal classes of the elementary schools" (p. 37). In 1942, Ramer followed 389 boys and 237 girls, now aged 25 to 37, from these classes; 73 percent were 25 to 30. Their IQ's in school, which ranged from 55 to 109, averaged 77, and most had IQ's between 70 and 84. All children had been tested "according the Binet-Simon method." As controls, Ramer chose 361 males and 228 females from Stockholm elementary schools in Stockholm and its suburbs, matching only on birth date. His aim was to compare special class cases with cases "largely representing the average citizen" (p. 41).

The following results are drawn from the author's summary:

1. Those with MR, more often than the comparisons, came from lower social classes and more had lost parents by death.
2. Males with MR had a higher mortality rate and a lower frequency of marriage. (Ramer suggested that it may be easier for a woman with MR to marry than for a man with MR: "This is quite a plausible explanation when we remember that, thanks to their primitive and uninhibited disposition, such women sometimes attract really quite normal men" [p. 82].)
3. Those with MR had more divorces.
4. The males with MR more often held "unqualified" jobs.
5. Those with MR more often received relief payments from the state. This was less frequent for individuals with an IQ of 85 and over.
6. More of those with MR needed mental care in institutions of different kinds.

7. No differences were found between those with MR and controls "as regards types of crime and relapses into crime" (p. 132). Ramer noted that results from previous studies he reviewed indicated that the intensity, extent, and degree of deficiency was in inverse proportion to the criminality, did not seem to apply to the cases investigated here. Nor did the figures presented bear out . . . other results showing that it was primarily those from the special class with higher IQ's who were most liable to turn criminal (p. 119).

Ramer's study was conducted when he was working at the State Institute of Human Genetics and Race Biology in Stockholm, and shows the explicit influence of eugenics.

The last of the four studies, carried out by Kennedy (1948), was reported in *The Social Adjustment of Morons in a Connecticut City.* Although the influence of eugenics is not apparent in Kennedy's report, the children who were followed up were selected from among "socially inadequate and individually handicapped persons" identified in 1937 by field workers trained at the Eugenics Record Office established by Davenport for the study of family stocks. The criteria used in the selection procedure were not stated. A later study by the same organization in 1944 classified some of those identified in 1937 as "morons,[2] defined by an IQ test rating between 45 and 75 . . . mostly children of school age who were living in their own homes with their parents or relatives." Kennedy selected a single community within the state where the 1937 census showed there were 260 "morons." To correct for possible omissions in the census, Kennedy checked the special class enrollment, and located fifteen additional persons. Fifty-nine percent of all study subjects had IQ's in the 65 to 75 range, and of these, 29 percent had IQ's of 70 to 75.

Kennedy described the nonretarded subjects as follows: "Inclusion of the . . . [controls] was considered to be essential, because it was felt that an estimate of the social and economic adjustment of morons would be meaningful and valid only if their records were matched, in every particular, against those of non-morons with approximately the same social and economic backgrounds and status" (p. 6). Matching was on age, sex, country of birth, nationality, and father's oc-

2. The author refers to the study subjects as "morons," but in her later follow-up of the same subjects she uses the term "mentally deficient."

cupation. Having matched for every MR subject, Kennedy eventually used only a 50 percent random sample of "controls" because of budget constraints. Despite the attempt to match on father's occupation, somewhat fewer of the fathers of the subjects with MR were engaged in jobs in upper occupational levels.

Kennedy summarized the adjustment of the two study groups:

> More of the morons who are unemployed are not working because of physical difficulties; fewer of them are students; more of them are in laboring occupations; more of them have changed jobs four to seven times; fewer of them are given higher ratings of work performance by their employers, and correspondingly more of them receive lower ratings; fewer of them are saving money, and fewer of them have telephones.

Kennedy also found that more of the families of origin of the subjects with MR received relief from government and social agencies (p. 66), and more had court records. There were no differences between the young adults with MR and their comparisons in age at time of marriage or numbers of their children. Somewhat more of those with MR were married, and more were divorced and had step- or adopted children; more had records of arrests, with more dispositions or penalties attached to their arrests. In leisure activities, the females with MR less often attended movies or went dancing than their comparisons. Those with MR of both genders less often read newspapers, magazines, or books.

The study was conducted shortly after the end of World War II. During the war, fewer of those with MR served in the armed services: of those who served, 13 percent of the men with MR and 46 percent of the comparisons held the rank of sergeant or above. After the war, of those who served, none of those with MR and half of the comparisons used the veterans' educational aid provided by the G.I. Bill of Rights (Servicemen's Readjustment Act). Differences in service histories may also account for the greater frequency of marriage among those with MR, because more remained in civilian employment during the war years.

In her final summation, Kennedy stated: "Certainly the main result of our investigation is a demonstration of the social adequacy, *within limits,* of the morons we studied. In their humble way, most of them are worthy citizens who bear their share of the social burden and do nothing to threaten the welfare of society" (p. 98).

Kennedy (1966) carried out a further follow-up of the same study population. In the report of that study, Kennedy referred back to the earlier one: "The most significant finding of the 1948 study was the great congruence of the two groups in most areas of adjustment. It was possible to state that mildly retarded subjects and matched controls behave very similarly in a similar social environment" (p. 2). This evaluation reflects the influence of the more favorable conventional wisdom that emerged after World War II and is more optimistic than her evaluation in 1948.

Summary of Findings from the Four Studies

Family background. The families of the children from special schools were not randomly distributed across the social class or socioeconomic scales, but were overrepresented at the lower end of the range. There was also evidence of more family problems.

Self-support. A considerable proportion of the young people followed were self-supporting, without aid from human service agencies; however, more individuals from special schools than comparisons needed some form of help.

Job histories. Those from special schools who were employed held jobs requiring fewer skills than comparisons.

Trouble with the law. Those involved in delinquency and illegal behavior were far fewer than expected, but those from special schools got into more trouble than the comparisons.

Marriage. There was no agreement among the four studies on the proportion of those with and without mental retardation who were married at follow-up. There was agreement, with one exception, that among those with mental retardation, fewer males than females were married. The exception in the Kennedy study may have been the result of the timing of the study, shortly after World War II.

Divorce. A larger proportion of those with mental retardation were divorced than the comparisons.

Offspring. The two early studies of Fairbanks and Baller reported that those with mental retardation had more children than comparisons. Kennedy found no difference.

Service in the armed services. Kennedy found that fewer of those with mental retardation had been in the services; those that had, had lower ranks.

These findings are very different from the pessimistic conventional wisdom about mental retardation, although they show differences between young adults with and without mental retardation and do not support Kennedy's optimistic evaluation that "the mildly retarded subjects and matched controls behave very similarly in a similar social environment" (Kennedy 1966, p. 2).

Evaluating Study Design and Methods

An important reason for reviewing the four follow-up studies was to learn about design and methodological factors that would need to be taken into account in planning the present study. The review was based on several questions.

Who were the children studied? The available information on the children in the four studies was limited to IQ score and whether the child had been placed in special programs. Fairbanks gave a mean IQ for the three groups she studied as 61, 72, and 72 but noted that some of the children had IQ's in the high 80's and 90's. All received special training. Baller gave mean IQ's for the males and females of 60 and 59, respectively; all children had IQ's of 70 or less, and all had been in special classes. Ramer gave a mean IQ of 77 for his study population, with a range of 55 to 109; all had been in special classes. Kennedy reported an IQ range of 45 to 75, with 58 percent between 67 and 75; 36 percent of the children had never been in special classes and a further 33 percent had attended special classes for two years or less. The childhood IQ's of these study populations clustered predominantly at the upper end of the mild MR range and included children who, according to the current upper cutoff point of 70 to 75, would not meet the IQ criterion of mental retardation. There is no way of knowing how representative the children in the studies were of children in the mild MR IQ range of 50 to approximately 70, or what criteria were used in placing them in some form of special education. Information on the young adults as children is scant and IQ test data from other sources were used. Without a knowledge of all the children with mild MR in these communities, there was no way of determining which children with mild MR were and were not included in the studies.

How were the nonretarded comparisons selected? The only way to determine whether the young adults with mental retardation were similar to or different from those who did not have mental retardation was to compare the two groups. Some of the investigators used the term "controls," which in experimental science means that subjects and controls are similar in every respect except for the presence or absence of the factor being studied. In studies of life histories, however, this is clearly impossible. A more realistic goal is to match each person with MR with someone without MR who is similar on a few salient factors, such as age and sex. Because a person's upbringing is clearly influential in his or her adult life, similarity in social milieu during childhood is another salient matching factor. Without some matching procedure in selecting nonretarded persons for comparison, there is no way of knowing whether similarities and differences are due to mental retardation or to other factors.

Fairbanks selected comparisons from a general survey of so-called "normal" children in the study area. Eliminating siblings of those with mental retardation, she chose a random sample of the remaining children with IQ's of 90 and above. Baller matched on gender, age, and nationality of parents and drew from the records of over 20,000 students. Comparisons were restricted to children with IQ's between 100 and 120. Ramer selected comparisons matching only on age, and they were drawn as a random sample from the state elementary schools. This eliminated some of the children from well-to-do families whose children attended private schools. No lower IQ limit was set for comparisons.

No attempt was made to match children according to their social upbringing in any of these studies, although Baller found that those with mental retardation were heavily overrepresented in families with lower socioeconomic status. Later epidemiological studies of mild MR have repeatedly obtained the same finding (see Richardson and Koller 1994). We cannot tell, then, whether differences found in these studies stem from the presence or absence of mild MR, or from variations in the socioeconomic status of families.

In the selection of comparisons, Kennedy matched on sex, age, and parents' nationality and religion. She did not match on parent citizenship, and more of the comparisons' parents were U.S. citizens. The fathers' occupations were matched "in a general way." The classification of occupations shows that more comparison fathers held managerial positions, but the classification was not given in terms of levels of skill.

Baller, in addition to finding socioeconomic differences between the children with MR and the comparisons, also widely separated the IQ of those with MR from the comparisons by requiring all comparisons to have IQ's between 100 and 120. Because of these two features of the study, it might be expected that the differences between the two groups would be larger than in the other studies, and this appears to be so.

In addition to matching on age and gender, it seems evident, then, that the family backgrounds of the two groups should be as similar as possible.

What effect does the wider (or macro-) environment have on the study? The broader social and economic conditions that prevailed at the time of the study may affect the results. Fairbanks's study area enjoyed an economic boom during and after World War I. At the time of Baller's study, Lincoln, Nebraska, was undergoing an economic depression. Kennedy carried out her study in the transition from a wartime to a peacetime economy after World War II, during which there had been a greater disruption in the lives of the comparisons than of those with mental retardation. More of those with MR had stayed in civilian jobs throughout the war and had thus accumulated job seniority. Many of the comparisons had recently returned from the war, some were taking advantage of the educational aid offered by the government, and some were reentering the labor force. These conditions may account for some of the study results; for example, more of those with MR reported current employment and being married than the comparisons. In each of the U.S. studies, a sizable number of children came from immigrant families, and some had very limited knowledge of the English language. It is probable that this affected the children's language skills, which may have been an obstacle in taking IQ tests.

What forms of analysis were used in presenting results? Study results were presented in a series of tables showing frequency distributions for those with and without mental retardation on a large number of separate variables, such as level of job skill and marital status, which served to fragment the lives of these young adults. Because researchers made no connection between the fragments, the results did not provide a comprehensive view of how the various aspects of their daily lives were related to each other.

Although tables for the entire study population were given, occasionally subdivided by gender, further classifications of the population would have been enlightening; it would have been useful, for example, to differentiate between persons who were married or single and examine how their lives might vary. Finally, the studies focused on the study subjects as adults and did not relate outcomes to their histories as children.

A Different Approach

In 1967 Edgerton published a landmark study, *The Cloak of Competence* (reissued in 1993), which followed-up adults who had been released from an "MR institution." Along with his colleagues, he continued with a series of studies that further followed up the adults in *The Cloak of Competence* and other adults with a history of mental retardation (Edgerton 1984, 1991). The studies are different, both in conception and in approach, from the four studies reviewed above, which used responses to questionnaires, focused largely on the characteristics of those studied, used nonretarded comparisons, and compared how the responses of the two groups were distributed.

In these studies, Edgerton and his colleagues used a holistic and naturalistic approach based on anthropological and sociological methods. They stated three fundamental principles:

> (a) that phenomena be seen in their relevant context; (b) that these phenomena be seen not only through the observer's eyes, but [through] those of the subjects as well; and, (c) that reactive procedures be avoided at the same time that the investigator regards himself as a part of the phenomenon under investigation. (p. 3)

This approach includes the study of persons with mental retardation in a variety of settings and their interaction with nonretarded peers, which allowed some comparisons between those with and without mental retardation to be made.

Data for the studies were collected by means of participant observation and interviews, that were less structured than those in the studies reviewed earlier. Investigators spent time in the study subjects' homes and in other settings that they frequented. Results were qualitative more than quantitative and included case studies. The results were an important source of insights and provided valuable verbal pictures of individuals that were missing in the other studies.

A difficulty with the Edgerton studies is that they do not indicate how representative of those who disappeared from services his findings were and provide no systematic information on the variability of the study population in terms of what happens to them. Edgerton concluded from his research that the young adults with mild mental retardation were not accepted by members of nonretarded peer groups:

> they are set apart from their peers, principally by the same academic limitations that troubled them in school—reading, writing and numerical calculations. They are seen as handicapped by their parents and other nonretarded persons and they themselves feel limited, often painfully so . . . In general, women have their primary ties with other mentally retarded persons, and the sources of social support most often and reliably come from their families. (1994b, p. 5)

In pursuing the question of what happens to children with mental retardation who disappear from services, both approaches—the four earlier studies and the Edgerton studies—are needed.

Reviewers' Summaries of Follow-up Studies

In addition to our own review of selected studies, we searched out the conclusions of other reviewers about what happened to children with mental retardation who disappeared from services after leaving school.

> Mild subnormality appears to be a temporary incapacity characterized mainly by educational difficulties experienced at school. (Kushlick and Blunden 1974, p. 42)
>
> It is apparent . . . that even during the depression years, substantial numbers of mentally subnormal children were able, upon leaving school, to find jobs for themselves and live as self-supporting, socially competent members of society. (Tizard 1965, p. 506)
>
> the methodological flaws of individual studies have frequently been so serious as to make findings of very limited reliability and conclusions of highly restricted generalizability. (Windle 1962, p. 20)
>
> it may be necessary to redress the balance by correcting false ideas that exist at the present time. The unduly pessimistic outlook which characterized thinking in the twenties and thirties would seem to have been replaced in the sixties and seventies by a degree of optimism that is scarcely warranted from a careful examination of available evidence. (Jackson 1977 p. 280)

No clear consensus emerges. Gruenberg's (1964) two alternatives may be considered the extremes of the range of possibilities (see Chapter 2), and it would seem that no single generalization can provide an answer. These studies and reviews may each hold some part of the answer, although they do not acknowledge how the lives of those studied vary. As we have learned, the answer to Gruenberg's question is far more complex than the two simple alternatives he posed.

After following up Baller's study population to an older age, Miller (1965) recognized the complexity that must be taken into account in planning further studies:

> The longitudinal inquiry begun by Baller, . . . and followed up in the present study, provides evidence of the importance of considering the individuality of persons regardless of classification. Herein perhaps lies the most important implication of the study as a whole. Environmental factors, physical capacities, and human interactions affect the exceptionally complex intellectual growth and functioning of a person. The data in this longitudinal inquiry indicate that each of the subnormal subjects has had a unique combination of influences affecting his intellectual growth and social adjustment. In order to understand and to help such persons, all of these influences must be considered. Finally, to understand better the subnormal individual, one should see him as a unique person interacting in his perceptual environment and should avoid thinking of him as one of a mass within a single classification. (p. 195)

Several studies have looked at children from special classes at older ages. Ross et al. (1985) followed children born between 1921 and 1925 whose average age was 46 or 47 at time of follow-up. Kennedy (1966) continued to follow the children in her earlier study to ages 32 to 40. Both studies used comparisons who did not have MR. Because this is a later stage in the life course than our follow-up to age 22—the circumstances and conditions of life are different in early adulthood and middle age—we will not review these studies further.

Why Do Some Do Better Than Others?

What may account for different outcomes becomes an important question because of the heterogeneity of the lives of those adults with childhood histories of mental retardation who disappeared from MR services after school-leaving age. There are two ways of addressing this question. One is to ask what factors in childhood histories predict various aspects of adult histories. The other is to examine interrelationships among factors in the adult histories. Baller and Ramer examined this question briefly, but gave no evidence to support their statements.

Baller inquired into "the respects in which the mentally subnormal individuals who succeed in making a reasonably satisfactory adjustment differ from those who fail" (p. 191)."He defined as "well adjusted" those who were wholly self-supporting and had records clear of breaches of the law or of violations of accepted standard of ethics. (Minor offenses such as arrest for speeding were not charged against a subject's record.) It is not clear how he identified violations of accepted standards of ethics. He found that a higher proportion of married than single women were well adjusted, and that well-adjusted women were more often of better personal appearance and superior training in domestic responsibilities. He could not find any particular factors in men that were associated with being well-adjusted: "There does seem to be, however, a rather marked degree of patience with the very drab work surroundings on the part of an appreciable number of self-supporting men."

Ramer related some characteristics of some children to later adult functioning. He found a tendency for males who were criminal as adults, for example, to have been more moody and delinquent as children.

To examine why some young adults with MR do better than others, there is no need to use nonretarded comparisons. Ferguson and Kerr (1960) examined the relationship between the IQ of children at special schools in Glasgow, Scotland, and their later functioning in their early twenties. Comparing those with IQ's below and above 60, they found that fewer of those with the lower IQ's had married, and that males with higher IQ's were involved in more crime. In job histories, they found that those with IQ's below 60 were less often employed than those with IQ's above 60. For the latter group, there was no difference in level of job skill (p. 110).

Cobb (1972) published a comprehensive review on predictive assessment of adults with MR for social and vocational adjustment. On the relationship between earlier IQ and later functioning, he concluded that

> Measures of intellectual competence taken in childhood cannot be assumed to describe intellectual competence in the adult years . . . The probability of finding IQ or similar measures to be predictively related to criteria of adult adjustment is a function of the intelligence range of the population sampled: the narrower the range, the less likely intelligence will be found significantly discriminating. (pp. 145, 146)

He commented further

> . . . that no simple formula for prediction is possible, that the relationships between predictors and criteria are enormously complex, and that outcomes in terms of personal, social and vocational success are the product of manifold interactive determinants. (p. 138)

In order to examine what childhood factors predict different adult histories, it is necessary to have systematic and comprehensive data on childhood histories. No study has yet collected such data.

Studies of Children with Mental Retardation Who Continue in Services as Young Adults

Gruenberg (1964) estimated that approximately one half of all children with mental retardation continued to receive some mental retardation services after school-leaving age. While there has been a large body of research literature on adults in different kinds of MR services, these studies did not initially select children and then follow them into adult services.

Almost all children with severe MR require continuing support and supervision after school-leaving age. Some are placed in MR institutions as children and continue there as adults. (For a review of studies of children and young people in institutions, see Richardson 1984.) Institutional policies and practices so govern the lives of these young people that they have little control over their lives. The past thirty years have seen a major shift away from institutional care, and earlier studies of institutions have little relevance today. Increasingly, care is provided within the communities where the children were brought up, including various forms of day services and support to the families.

There is little systematic information about children with mild MR who receive MR services as adults, or how much time they spend in services and what kind of services they receive. Further, little is known about their daily lives as adults, or what distinguishes those adults with mild MR who receive services and those who do not.

We found one study that followed up on children with more severe mental retardation. Saenger's (1957) study population had been brought up in New York City. He posed a number of questions about their lives as adults: "Do they prove to be serious problems to their families; do they make a satisfactory adjustment among their neighbors and friends; can they hold some kind of a job, sheltered or competitive; or do they become a well-defined social problem with possible conflict with the law?" (p. xv). Because of severe mental retardation it was expected that the study subjects would continue to require sheltering, support, and supervision after leaving school. To examine this did not require study of nonretarded persons for comparison.

On residential care, Sanger found that 26 percent of the sample were resident in institutions, 14 percent were now living in the community but had formerly been in institutions, and 52 percent had never been in institutions; 8 percent had died. Institutional placement usually occurred either during the school years or shortly after, and was due to changes in the family, such as the aging and death of parents. These placements were more frequent in broken homes and families marked by low cohesion, and there was a high correlation between institutionalization and the child's behavior problems.

Among those who lived at home as adults, Saenger found that

1. 76 percent had at least one additional disability. The most common were speech impediments, vacant facial expression, and faulty coordination.
2. their ability to communicate influenced their interaction with their families: half were able to communicate with their families in a limited way; a quarter were able to take an animated interest in the life of the family, were occasionally concerned with the problems of others, and tried to help where they could.
3. three quarters of the parents felt their child was easy to get along with.
4. family tension and parental rejection characterized the families of adults with more severe problems.
5. the adults spent a major portion of their time by themselves,

most often listening to the radio and watching TV, or doing nothing.

6. nearly one half regularly helped with household chores.
7. they often participated in activities such as visiting relatives and friends and attending movies and ballgames only with family members.
8. any friendships were of a strictly limited nature.

Implications for the Present Study

For adults who received MR services, these services were an important influence in their lives. Because they received services, they were more readily available for research purposes. In planning the present study, we recognized that the children with MR who disappeared from services after leaving school would have more complex adult histories than those who were in services. Some of those who disappeared might have had histories similar to peers who did not have mental retardation. For them, a wide range of data dealing with various facets of daily life, such as their marital histories, children, job histories, activities engaged in outside of working hours, and their own perception of their lives, would be needed.

4

Setting, Design, and Methods

The Setting of the Study

The city of Aberdeen is situated between two rivers, the Dee and the Don, on the northeast coast of Scotland. It is seventy miles from Dundee and stands apart from other large towns and cities. Its agricultural and forested hinterland stretches west about forty miles to the Grampian Mountains.

The history of Aberdeen dates back to the twelfth century, and it became an early trading center. Robert Bruce granted the town several charters of rights, including the Great Charter, in 1319. Its greatest growth, however, occurred in the nineteenth century, when granite quarrying became an important local industry and the harbor facilities were developed. The availability of these facilities encouraged the expansion of steamship service, deep sea fishing, and ship building and repair. The extension of railway lines to Aberdeen also helped to transform the city into a transportation center, from which fish and agricultural products could to be sent south to markets in the United Kingdom. At this time there was a major development of roads and new buildings in the city, many of the latter constructed of local granite.

In the 1960s and 1970s, the period of the present study, the population of Aberdeen ranged from approximately 180,000 to 185,000. There were approximately 3,000 births each year, with some drop occurring after 1962. The five birth cohorts of 1951 to 1955 used in the present study included 13,842 children. The population was predominantly comprised of families who had lived in Scotland for many generations. A small minority had come from other parts of the United Kingdom, but there were no ethnic or foreign national minority groups who might have been the focus of prejudice and discrimination, or whose first language was other than English. This was an advantage, because the study of mental retardation was not confounded by minority group status or language differences.

The economy of Aberdeen was diverse. Local industries included manufacture of machinery, various textiles, and paper; marketing and processing of agricultural products; building; tailoring; and rose-growing. During the period of the study, the fishing industry, along with shipbuilding and repairing, was declining. Aberdeen was a railroad, air, and sea transportation center. Tourism was important; summer visitors benefited from the city's recreational facilities and used Aberdeen as a convenient point of access to the coastal scenery, historical sites, and recreational facilities in the northeast of Scotland. The city also served as a shopping and medical center for the surrounding area.

In 1971, British Petroleum announced large oil finds in the North Sea, and the development of oil and natural gas production had a major impact on Aberdeen, which developed into the main administrative, service, supply, and communications center for the industry in the United Kingdom. Most of the offshore and onshore jobs were filled by in-migrants with previous experience in the oil business, or by older local men with experience in similar industries. The oil industry offered only a few job opportunities for local young adults at the time of our study.

The University of Aberdeen, which included a medical school and a college of education, was an important center of higher education and research. Commercial and technical colleges, as well as several research institutes, were also located in the city.

A number of city agencies provided services for the study population and their families. The director of the Department of Education was responsible for overseeing the welfare of all school-age children in both municipal and private schools. The presence of a single administrative authority proved a great benefit to the study, because department records covered all children, including those who had, for whatever reason, been placed outside of Aberdeen. The department provided special educational services for all children with disabilities, including mental retardation.

Aberdeen had great civic pride and valued education. Over 30 percent of the tax base contribution to the cost of governing the city was devoted to the education service. At the time of the study, there were several city-supported nursery schools for children aged 2 to 5 years. These schools were intended to provide close personal care, medical supervision, and informal training, both mental and social. Attendance was voluntary. Compulsory education began at age 5, and children attended primary schools until about the age of 12. From then on, until a minimum of age 15 to 16, children were educated in secondary school. There were also senior secondary schools designed primarily for children going on to higher education. Most were non-fee-paying and under the direct management of the Education Authority, but some were independent private schools. (For a description of the special educational program, see Chapter 15.)

The city health department was under the direction of the medical officer of health. The Health Visitor Service was, by statute, responsible for visits at regular intervals to preschool children in their homes. Health visitors assessed the health of the infants and the conditions of child care, discussed the care of the child with the mother, reported problems that required medical attention, and arranged for vaccinations and immunizations. The School Health Service provided routine medical evaluations at ages 5, 9, and 13 as a statutory requirement, and audiometric and vision screening tests. School doctors were available, at the request of parents or teachers, for special examinations of children. The Department of Health was also responsible for children with mental retardation in residential care at facilities in Aberdeen. A Child Guidance Clinic offered evaluation and treatment for children with behavior disturbance.

A close cooperative relationship existed between the Departments of Education and Health. The school medical officer worked closely with school authorities in evaluating children with disabilities and disorders. Their help in the present study was invaluable in many ways.

At the time the study subjects were in school, the Department of Social Work had assigned social workers who understood the problems related to mental retardation to the special schools. They knew all the children in the schools and their families, and often maintained contact after the young people left school. As the study population grew older, the policies of the Department of Social Work changed. Social workers were assigned to specific areas of the community rather than to particular schools. Because of the change, young people with MR and the social workers whom they had grown to know had less ongoing contact and fewer continuing relationships.

The local authorities had responsibility for the care and welfare of children whose parents were unable to provide for them. Children were placed in a reception center to determine their needs and the most appropriate form of care. The available alternatives were residential homes, foster parents, and for adolescents, a hostel. Several study children had been placed in these facilities.

The National Health Service Act of 1947 established regional boards to administer hospitals, and because medical care was financed on a national basis, individuals were not required to pay for services. This development was important for the study because it was unnecessary to consider financial differences in access to medical care as a factor in the histories of the study population.

In 1958, the local government established a Department of Housing Management, which was responsible for all dwellings built by the City Corporation. Between 1919 and 1958, the Corporation constructed over 16,000 housing units on a number of housing estates within the city. During the same period, the Scottish Special Housing Association built approximately 1,800 housing units. By 1970, the number of municipally owned housing units was approximately equal to that in private ownership. Many of the young people in the study and their families lived in these municipal housing units. An impetus for building municipal housing was the severe substandard conditions of the old tenements. Some were demolished and others renovated.

A comprehensive network of local bus services was widely used in the city and surrounding community in 1962, when data were collected for the Birch et al. (1970) study; by the late 1970s, however, the large increase in the use of cars had resulted in a corresponding decrease in bus service. The city offered a wide variety of recreational facilities, including parks, gardens, and beaches; sports facilities for bowling, putting, golf, soccer, rugby, and cricket; children's playgrounds; public libraries and museums; a theater, a concert hall, and movie houses; places to dance; and numerous pubs, bars, and restaurants. The use of the outdoor facilities was seasonal: in summer, it remained light most of the night; in winter the days were very short, and the weather often inclement. By the 1970s, television had become an important part of daily life.

The Feasibility of a Follow-up Study

To determine whether or not to undertake a follow-up study, we took two initial steps: First, we discussed the proposed study with all the people in Aberdeen whose interest and cooperation were essential—city officials responsible for the various forms of records and the faculty of various departments at the University of Aberdeen who had relevant experience and knowledge. Richardson knew many of them from the Birch et al. (1970) study. Second, we ascertained the extent to which the study population could be traced at age 22, and whether they and their parents would be willing to cooperate in the study. We selected a random sample of the young people with MR and, of these, traced 82 percent. We judged that a more exhaustive search for the remaining 18 percent would in fact locate many of them. Using a sample of young people classified as mentally retarded in childhood who had been born prior to the study cohorts, we began pretest interviewing, and it was clear that a large proportion were willing to be interviewed. Based on this work, we decided to undertake the follow-up study.

Selecting Young People for the Study

Children with Mental Retardation

To the three birth cohorts of children with MR in the original study (1952, 1953, 1954), it was necessary to add two additional birth cohorts (1951 and 1955). This increased the number of children in the study from 104 to 221, the minimum required, in our estimation, to carry out the analyses we envisioned. The increase was more than twofold because a number of children in the three original cohorts were not classified as having MR until after the earlier study was conducted and thus were missed.

Our follow-up study used the same definition of mental retardation as the earlier study (see Chapter 1) and the same methods to identify all children who fit the definition. The total number of children born between 1951 and 1955 and resident in Aberdeen in 1962 was 13,842. (In Chapter 5, this number is used as the denominator in determining prevalence.) Of the 221 young people with MR from the five birth cohorts for the present study, 10 had died by age 22. Of the 211 survivors, data for 15 were incomplete because both parent and young adult refused to participate, and for 3 others because we were unable to trace them. Thus, the numbers included in the different analyses we present in this book vary, depending on the data needed. In the prevalence analyses (Chapter 5), for example, all 221 subjects were included; in the etiology analyses, the numbers come close to 221; in analyses that required interview data, the numbers were lower.

Comparisons

In order to examine the similarities and differences between the young people with MR and nonretarded peers, we selected comparisons from a one-in-five random sample of all children who were born in the same years as the subjects and resided in Aberdeen in 1962. The requirements for selection were that no comparison had ever been placed in a mental retardation facility or scored below 75 on either of two group intelligence tests given to all children in the city at ages 7 and 9. For each person with MR, we chose a comparison who was matched for age, gender, area of residence in the city, and social class of the head of the household in which the child lived. In the earlier study, lower social class and an undesirable area of residence were overrepresented among families of children with MR. Because of this skewing, social class and area of residence were used as matching variables to obtain a similar social milieu during childhood for the children with MR and comparisons.

We were unable to interview all the comparisons selected in this manner. Some we could not locate, some did not wish to be interviewed, and following those who had moved away from Aberdeen would have been costly. We were able to collect data on 75 percent of all the original comparisons chosen. For the remaining 25 percent, we selected alternates who had the same matching characteristics as the original comparisons.

Children in Regular Classes with IQ's in the Mild MR Range

To identify children whose IQ fell within the mild MR range, although they had never been classified as MR, we selected all children in the birth cohorts 1951–1955 with scores below 75 on both of the group IQ tests given at ages 7 and 9 who remained in regular schools. These children are sometimes referred to as "borderline" subjects.

Tracing Subjects

We used a wide variety of methods to trace the young adults. School records provided the names and addresses of parents during the school years, and we successfully traced many of the subjects through their parents, who supplied their children's current addresses. If parents had moved since their child left school, we searched for their names in telephone books, current voting registers, and records of the local authorities. When this was unsuccessful, we made inquiries among the neighbors and local shops where they used to live. We also sought out family relatives.

Subjects in adult MR services were traced through the records kept by the service providers. In some cases, the family doctor knew current addresses. If young women had married, we searched for their married names in the local newspaper announcements and in the marriage registries. In a few cases, we located subjects when they placed their child's birth announcement in the newspaper; the paper provided the address of the person submitting the announcement. If this was a relative, we asked the relative for the subject's address.

In most cases the process was relatively simple. For some, however, tracking took a great deal of time, ingenuity, and even luck. We learned that many of those who had moved away from Aberdeen returned to the city to visit family and friends; where possible, we interviewed them when they visited. In these ways, we were able to trace 98 percent of the study population.

New Research Data

General Considerations

The follow-up was carried out when the young people reached the age of 22. By that age, they had had approximately seven years of postschool experience. For those who disappeared from MR services after leaving school, this provided an amount of time sufficient to determine how well they functioned in the various roles expected of young adults by society.

To collect data for all the study subjects at age 22 required a five-year time span, the span covered by their births. We conducted interviews with the parents of each study subject and then, independently, with the study subjects themselves, for several reasons:

- The parent and young adult would each be in a better position to provide specific types of information. In general, the parents were better able to provide histories on the upbringing and earlier years of their child. The young people not in MR services knew more about their own histories for the period from age 16 to 22, the postschool years.
- The same data were obtained from both parent and young adult for the main outline of the study subjects' lives, which provided a cross-check on the data obtained.
- For the young adults with severe MR who were unable to provide the needed data, the parents were asked to do so.
- If, for any reason, we were unable to interview the young adults, the parent interview provided information needed for the study.

The parent interview was generally with the mother, but at times the father was also present. When it was not possible to interview the mother due to refusal, death, or other reasons, we interviewed the father. When neither parent was available, we interviewed another family member, an adult who had been a surrogate parent, a relative, or a member of the staff of the residential institutions were the young person lived. From the pretest interviews with the young adults and their parents, we learned what kinds of questions and language they best understood and became familiar with their use of local dialect and vocabulary. (Stephen Richardson, who grew up in Scotland, had some knowledge of the local idioms and to some extent could use them when appropriate.)

At the outset of the study, we did not know how much of the data we sought could be elicited from young adults with varying degrees of severity of MR or what methods were most appropriate in interviewing them. Throughout the range of mild MR, we were able to obtain comprehensive life histories from the young adults using the methods described below. We were also able to obtain partial histories from some of the young adults with severe MR. In a number of cases, when we interviewed young adults in their parents' home, the parents told us beforehand that their child would not be interviewable. They expressed great surprise when the interview lasted two hours or more and their child was forthcoming and communicative. In general, we found that the ability of these young adults to talk about their lives had been underestimated.

Development of the Interviews

Using the pretest population born in 1950, we carried out pilot interviews. The initial interviews were exploratory, guided by a general set of topics rather than a prepared set of questions. These served as conceptual pigeonholes into which we could slot responses, and, as one might expect, their number increased as we learned more about the lives of these young people. In this way we developed the first draft of a standardized interview, which then went through several revisions, each used in a series of trial interviews, before reaching its final form.

One ongoing task was to organize the interview and frame the questions in order to elicit the data we sought and to arrange the questions in a sequence most effective in meeting the interview objectives. Interviews were restricted to the time informants were willing to give, yet they had to cover the range of information we sought. Once their cooperation and interest had been secured, informants were generally willing to continue for two or three hours. The amount of time spent on each interview varied according to the talkativeness of the informants and the complexity of their histories. We tried to restrict the interview to a single session, but on some occasions we continued in a second session if the informant was willing.

In arranging the sequence of questions for each section of the interview, we would begin with factual and descriptive information and leave the potentially more sensitive or threatening questions until later. We concluded each section with a less threatening task by asking the informant to evaluate the information he or she had just given. We tried to vary the pace of the interview and in places asked questions informants generally enjoyed answering; at the end of the section on schooling, for example, we asked, "If you had been running the school, what changes would you have made to make it a better school for you?" If we found that what informants were saying was inconsistent or contradictory, we tried to resolve the differences. At the end of each interview we asked informants how they felt about the interview and how they would evaluate it. Their comments and suggestions were useful in planning changes that would be beneficial.

In the pretests we attempted to find informants with widely diverse life histories. For the young adults who had more severe difficulties with comprehension and communication, we adapted the interview to elicit any relevant information they could give us. The exploratory interviews and the development of the final standardized interview format were carried out by Stephen Richardson with the help of a research assistant, Janice McLaren.

In the preliminary interviews we learned how to explain the purpose of the study to the informant. We included this explanation in an introductory letter, in our phone calls to make an appointment for the interview, and at the beginning of the interview itself. No reference was made to mental retardation, and informants were encouraged to ask questions about any concerns they might have.

Throughout the study we remained flexible about the interview location. We offered informants the option of being interviewed in their homes or at an office at the university. If an informant preferred to come to the university, the interviewer would, if the informant wished, provide transportation. Some informants in adult MR services were interviewed at the service facility. Others, who had attended the special school but had subsequently disappeared from services and married without telling their spouses that as children they had been classified as mentally retarded, chose to be interviewed in the research office in order to avoid disclosing that part of their history. The majority of the study interviews took place in the general vicinity of Aberdeen. Informants living in other parts of the United Kingdom were interviewed, when possible, during a return visit to Aberdeen. For the remainder, interviewers traveled to the areas where the young people lived. Some had emigrated from the United Kingdom, and for two of these, Richardson obtained a parent interview in Canada. The methods used in the developing the parent interview were similar to those used for the young adult interview.

Several of the research subjects were very difficult to contact: they were away at sea, for example, or they worked unpredictable or irregular hours, or they were involved with social, health, or domestic problems. Some had a poor sense of time and would forget appointments, or were so elusive and evasive that it took many visits and a disproportionate amount of the interviewer's time before an interview was obtained.

All interviews, including the pilot interviews, were tape-recorded. In every case, permission was requested, and no one objected once the interviewer had explained our reasons for needing the recording and assured confidentiality.

The tape recordings served two important purposes. They enabled the interviewers to give full attention to the interview. This freed them from the task of writing down more than a few notes during the actual interview and allowed them to complete the write-up later from the tape recording. The recordings also provided a basis for evaluating the methods used by the interviewers and checking on the accuracy and completeness of the write-up.

In developing the interview format we kept two important considerations in mind: first, the time and effort invested at this point were worthwhile, because no amount of analytical expertise or sophistication could turn poor data into sound results; second, the particular set of circumstances and conditions provided a research opportunity that was unique and exciting but also fraught with hazard. The study required steering a careful course between the Scylla of trying to obtain too much information, thus losing the cooperation of informants, overburdening interviewers, and amassing a body of data that would not be fully analyzed, and the Charybdis of being so limited and specific in the research design that this unusual opportunity was inadequately exploited. Our concern was to hold to a middle course.

Form of the Final Interviews

Content

The interview had to be flexible in construction in order to cover the informants' widely varying life histories. We tried to avoid questions that might be painful, offensive, or simply irrelevant. The interview consisted of a set of core questions that were asked of all respondents and then, depending on their responses, further optional questions. Once the marital status was obtained, for example, separate sets of questions were used for those who were single, married, separated,

Table 4.1a Parent interview

Core questions asked all parents	Optional questions asking for detailed information stemming from responses to core questions
Family census Question about family members Mother's pregnancy losses Others living in household	Children who were adopted, step, or foster
Chronology of places lived for parents and young adult	Each past and present residence in any institution Present home of young person, whether still with parents or elsewhere, such as with spouse
Education history of young adult Parent's evaluation of education young adult received	Nursery school Regular school Special school or Junior Occupation Center,[a] including reasons sent Home, no schooling
Chronology of post-school occupational career (age 16–22)	Jobs Periods unemployed Attending MR day center
Assessment of job experiences	Homebound (not seeking work) Housewife
Health Interests Social relationships	
Marital status	Opposite-sex relationship for singles Marital relationship Unmarried mothers
Upbringing of young adult Aspirations for young adult Conclusions	Problems and rewards parent experienced

a. See Chapter 5 for definitions.

divorced, and widowed. The topics covered in both the core and optional sections in the parent and young adult interviews are shown in summary form in Tables 4.1a and 4.1b. This arrangement enabled interviewers to tailor the interview to the specific history of each individual.

Table 4.1b Young adult interview

Core questions asked all young adults	Optional questions asking for detailed information stemming from responses to core questions
Chronology of places lived	Each past and present residence in any institution Present home, whether still with parents or elsewhere, such as with spouse
Education history Evaluation of education	Regular school, special school, or Junior Occupation Center[a]
Chronology of post-school occupational career (age 16–22) Past and present occupations Evaluation of occupational career	Jobs Periods unemployed, further education, training, attending MR day center, homebound (not seeking work), part-time jobs, housewife (present occupation explored extensively)
Marital status	Single, married, divorced/separated, widowed Unmarried mothers Children
Health Interest and activities Social relationships	
Level of functioning Aspirations Conclusions	

a. See Chapter 5 for definitions.

Alternative Forms of the Interview Schedules

In the course of the interviewing, we found it necessary to develop alternative forms of the interview schedules. Some informants were unwilling to give the time needed for the full schedule but did agree to a brief interview. Rather than lose the opportunity to interview them, we developed a shortened interview that contained demographic information and a chronological summary of their life histories. The shortened interview was used with 3 percent of the parents and 5 percent of the young adults.

In some cases, following an attempt at the full interview, it became apparent that informants either had difficulty understanding the questions or were very limited in their responses. For them we developed a simplified schedule, which we used for 16 percent of all the young adults with MR. An additional 8 percent were so limited in speech that no formal interview was possible.

Because some study subjects lived in inaccessible places, we developed a mail questionnaire to obtain the main outline of their histories.

Types of Questions Used

Our purpose was to use interview questions that were as simple and understandable as possible in a form that would be congenial to the thought processes and language usage of the respondents. In this way, we increased the likelihood that we would gain the information we sought. The basic principles and methods used in the interviews were based on *Interviewing: Its Forms and Functions* (Richardson, Dohrenwend, and Klein 1965).

We considered incorporating some of the scales and tests available in the early 1970s and relevant to the study purposes, and even tried out a few in the development of the interview, but we found them unsuitable. The informants had difficulty understanding the questions; they disliked the large number of short-answer questions; and the scales took up a disproportionate amount of time in an interview that necessarily covered a wide range of content.

In considering the form of questions to use, we also had to consider the subsequent analysis of the data. Questions calling for a response the interviewer could place in prearranged categories would facilitate analysis. These generally took the form of closed questions requiring only short responses such as yes or no, choosing from a set of alternatives, or giving specific information, such as age. Wherever appropriate, we used this question form, but when the response was yes, we asked a follow-up question to ascertain the validity of the response, and this often elicited useful information. If, for example, an informant answered yes to the question "Do you have any friends where you work?," the interviewer would then ask for descriptions of the friends and what they did together.

Informants with intellectual limitations often had difficulty understanding and responding to questions that asked them to choose from a series of alternative responses, especially if the alternatives were abstractions. We found we had to use more open-ended questions than we would have used for informants with normal intelligence.

Open questions required responses longer than a few words. To learn about leisure-time activities, for example, we asked informants what they had done during the previous weekend; follow-up probes asked for specifics or for more information on periods of the weekend not covered in the initial response. Open questions enabled us to obtain information in a form chosen by, and congenial to, the thought patterns and speech usage of the informants and increased the quality and validity of the responses. But this gain in information was achieved at the price of then having to perform content analyses and develop categories in order to quantify the responses. We recognized that using open questions and further probing required a high level of interview skill.

The Write-up of the Interview

According to study procedures, the interviewers were to listen to the tape recording and enter the information called for by the interview schedule. Because they were encouraged to speak freely, respondents' answers sometimes included valuable unsolicited information sought in other questions. When this occurred, the interviewer cross-referenced the unsolicited response to the appropriate questions.

To have transcribed the entire interview would have been prohibitive both in time and in cost, yet some responses were of sufficient importance to warrant full transcription by a typist. In selecting sections of the tape for transcription, we looked for examples of insights that threw light on specific research issues, as well as other important issues related to mental retardation not included in the study research designs, and passages that described something in a way that was so vivid or moving, the verbatim transcription contributed to our understanding. These transcriptions became part of the record of the interview.

Selecting and Training Interviewers

When the final forms of the young adult and parent interviews were completed, and Richardson and McLaren had gained experience in conducting and writing up the interview, we selected and trained a team of interviewers. To reduce inconsistencies that might result from having interviewers of both sexes and different ages, we selected women who were around thirty years of age. This made it unlikely that they would be identified as peers by either the parents or the young adults.

Because of the special nature of these interviews, we preferred selecting as interviewers individuals who had no previous experience in interviewing. We based our selection largely on an assessment of the applicant's experience and skill in interpersonal relations and a prior history of good job performance. Most of the interviewers had been teachers, and one had been a psychiatric nurse. In addition to Richardson and McLaren, eight other interviewers worked on the project. Given the demanding nature of the work, the turnover was remarkably low, which was beneficial in developing a team of experienced, highly skilled workers and reducing training costs. Our experience showed that full-time interviewing was emotionally, physically, and intellectually taxing, and it was preferable to have interviewers work only part-time. Since many of them had children, they found the possibility of part-time work attractive.

Once hired, trainee interviewers were given intensive instruction in the purposes of the research, the content and organization of the interview, interviewing techniques, and a general orientation to the issue of mental retardation and the organization of services in Aberdeen. Then as observers they accompanied previously trained interviewers on a parent interview and young adult interview. Trainees then reviewed and discussed the experience with the trained interviewers. In the next step of the training, the trainees interviewed each other and then carried out practice interviews with selected parents and young adults. (These were families we had already interviewed for our research who had expressed an interest in helping us.) For the first of their interviews, McLaren accompanied the trainees. When the trainee was able to do an interview adequately, she conducted a practice interview alone and wrote up the interview. Then McLaren reviewed the tape recording and write-up in detail and discussed them with the trainee. Only when the trainee had reached a satisfactory level of performance did she begin interviewing new study subjects.

To ensure the confidentiality of data, interviewers were instructed in a set of procedures. Each subject was given a number. Then the face sheet of the interview, which matched the number to the name and address, was removed to a locked file. Thereafter, the interview was identified by number only and kept in separate locked files. The tape recordings, also identified by number alone, were stored in a locked cabinet in a separate building. During training, interviewers were reminded of their responsibility for maintaining confidentiality, including never discussing the content of interviews with anyone except project staff.

Throughout the data gathering, McLaren and sometimes also Richardson held regular meetings with the interviewers to share experiences and discuss any problems they encountered. Because interviewers were not allowed to discuss their work with anyone except research staff, these meetings met important emotional and intellectual needs.

Interviewers were also trained to use the observations schedule. When the trainee accompanied a more experienced interviewer on an interview, each filled in separate schedules and later compared and discussed them. This procedure was also followed when trainees interviewed informants who had already been interviewed.

Quality Control of Interview Data

The development, standardization, and quality control of the interviewing proceeded in three steps.

1. *During development of the interview.* Richardson carried out the early pilot interviews and developed a draft of content areas. McLaren, the first assistant for the study taken on in Aberdeen, accompanied Richardson on his interviews, and later they discussed each interview in terms of method and content. McLaren conducted interviews on her own, and afterwards wrote up the interviews from the tape recording. Both Richardson and McLaren then reviewed the tape recording and write-up.

2. *After formal interviewing started.* When additional interviewers had been hired and trained, Richardson and McLaren then jointly reviewed the methods, content, and write-up of each interview for the first six months of the study while listening to the tape recording. At this point, McLaren became interview supervisor and coordinator.

3. *After the first six months of formal interviewing.* A research assistant read through each of the written interviews, checking that all ques-

tions had been answered, there were no discrepancies or ambiguities, and there was consistency in the data where cross-checks were available. If this editing check revealed sections needing additions or clarifications, the write-up was returned to the interviewer for this purpose.

Each interviewer, in turn, took time off from interviewing to monitor selected interviews of her colleagues. She listened to the tape recording and reviewed the write-up of the interview, paying particular attention to whether the written record accurately reflected the tape recording and whether there were any omissions in the write-up or errors in the techniques and methods used during the interview. The person responsible for monitoring then met with McLaren, and later with the interviewer, to review her evaluation. Each interviewer, at different times, took turns being reviewer and critic, and in this way they learned from one another. This procedure helped maintain standard interview methods, and the quality and accuracy of the interview write-ups.

Observations

At the completion of each interview, the interviewer filled in an observation schedule on aspects of the informant's appearance, manner, behavior, use and comprehension of language, dress, and cleanliness. Observations about the home setting were also recorded, if the interview took place there, and whether other people were present during the interview. Table 4.2 gives an outline of the observations.

Documentary Sources

Many documentary sources provided data for the study. These included data that had been initially collected for other research purposes in Aberdeen as well as administrative records maintained by local, health, education, social work, and judicial authorities.

Data Collected for Other Research Purposes

Data collected for the earlier study. Several different types of data were collected for the Birch et al. (1970) study:

Table 4.2 Observations

Location of interview
Description of the building, the room in which the interview took place, and the general condition of the room, that is, whether it was untidy, dirty, or smelly.

Description of informant
1. Height, weight, facial characteristics, other bodily features, movement, dress, personal hygiene, speech, vision, and hearing.
2. Vocabulary, comprehension of interview questions, quality of responses, and general attentiveness of the informant.

Informant's attitude during the interview
Scales of outgoing to withdrawn, relaxed to tense, friendly to hostile, evidence of a sense of humor, and whether the informant showed any unusual display of emotion.

1. Obstetrical and neonatal
2. Wechsler Intelligence Scale for Children
3. Results of the pediatric neurological examination
4. Results of the psychiatric assessment
5. The social class ratings of families in Aberdeen

(For the first four types of data, see Chapter 1, and for greater detail, Birch et al. 1970. For a description of social class, see Chapter 14.)

Survey of Mental Retardation in Northeast Scotland. In the 1970s, a research unit of the Medical Research Council, under the direction of Dr. George Innes, conducted a survey of mental retardation for northeast Scotland, including Aberdeen (Innes et al. 1978). The major emphasis of the survey was medical and it included the following data:

1. Cytogenetic examination and analysis
2. Medical history
3. Wechsler Adult Intelligence Scale
4. Goodenough Draw-a-Man
5. Vineland Social Maturity Scale
6. Holborn Reading Scale
7. Form of care being received at time of study
8. Summary social data on family, education, and occupation

Sixty-eight percent of the young people in the present study were covered by this survey. Those missed were largely individuals who received no MR services after leaving school.

Records from delinquency study. In the 1970s, Dr. David May, of the department of sociology at the University of Aberdeen, carried out a study of delinquency based on court records of the city of Aberdeen (May 1981). From these data, we could ascertain which of the study subjects were involved in court appearances and the disposition of cases.

Data Collected from Administrative Records

The administrative records we consulted varied in their completeness, standardization, and coverage of the study subjects. In general, records required for legal purposes tended to be in a more standard and complete form. In Aberdeen, which enjoyed a long tradition of close cooperation between officials and agencies of local government and researchers from the university, the production and storage of administrative records had received unusual attention. Government officials were aware of the potential research value of good administrative records, and the existence of a National Health Service and other human service agencies facilitated uniform record keeping.

Education records. For all the young adults in the study, there was a personal school record card listing attendance, level of performance in school work, reports of conduct and a medical card. All children in regular schools were given group intelligence tests at ages 7, 9, and 11. The scores for the subjects of the present study, which already had been used for research purposes, were available on computer tape. The intelligence test data were used to identify the "borderline" subjects. In addition, all information used in the decision to classify members of the study population as mentally retarded was available, including results of individual IQ tests. The school psychologist gave individual IQ tests to all children before they were classified as MR, using the Terman-Merrill revisions of the Stanford Binet Intelligence Scale. These tests were given at the time of the decision and periodically thereafter throughout the school years. The health services in Aberdeen are required by statute to give all children medical examinations at ages 5, 9, and 13. If needed, further special examinations are also carried out. The records of all these examinations for the study population were available to us.

Child guidance. A Child Guidance Center provided diagnostic and treatment services for children in Aberdeen and worked in close cooperation with the school authorities. The center's records for children in the present study were made available to us.

Social work. Three staff members from the Department of Social Welfare were responsible for maintaining a close liaison between the special schools and the homes of the study subjects throughout their time in special schools or residential care. These officials also acted as a liaison between the schools and other city agencies. The department served all the children in the city, including some of the comparison and borderline children in the study. Records of all contacts were maintained. The department was required by law to prepare background information for all juveniles who came in contact with the police and judicial system. Records of these reports and the disposition of each case were also made available to us.

Regional Hospital Board and Aberdeen Department of Health. Children's Hospital records were made available to us in order to obtain health histories of the study population. Dr. Keith Goulden reviewed these histories and also examined electroencephalography (EEG) records for all children who had been tested. (See Chapter 1 for a description of the health visitor records.) Officials of residential institutions for children and adults with MR kept systematic and detailed records of everyone under their care. They provided information on each individual's general history of care and medical history, programs in the institutions in which the individuals participated, periodic assessments of each person's level of functioning, and records of visitors they received and visits they made outside of the institution. These facilities were under the jurisdiction of the Regional Hospital Board and the Department of Health.

In addition to these data sources, we also referred to a comprehensive history of mental retardation services in the city (Forsyth et al. 1976).

In developing the study, we examined all these record sources and prepared data extraction forms. As a change of pace, interviewers carried out some record searches, but the administrative staff on the research project completed the majority of the work.

From these varied data sources we derived a number of measures for the present study (these measures are described in the chapters that document their use). IQ, however, a measure we used throughout the study, needs definition here.

IQ. Several IQ scores for each child, obtained at different ages, were available to us. Because we needed a single score for general classification, we decided to use the IQ scores recorded when the children were 8 to 10 years of age to be consistent with the 1962 study. For children born between 1952 and 1954, we used the scores on the Wechsler Intelligence Scale for Children (WISC) obtained by the team of American psychologists who were involved in the 1962 study and individually tested the children (Birch et al. 1970). For the remaining children, we used the scores in the Terman-Merrill revision of the Stanford-Binet Intelligence Scale or the Scottish Moray House Picture Test of Intelligence, administered by the Aberdeen School Psychologist. By comparing the WISC with the other scores for these children, we ascertained the difference between tests. For children not given the WISC, we adjusted the other test scores to give scores equivalent to the WISC. (See Chapter 7 for a discussion of the history of children's IQ scores during the school years.)

Part II

Epidemiology

5

Prevalence

In epidemiology, two terms are used to characterize the degree to which a disease or disorder is present in a population at risk. *Incidence* is the term used to describe the number of new cases arising in the population over a given period of time. *Prevalence* is the number of cases, old and new, known to exist at a particular point or over a given period of time. Incidence and prevalence are both expressed as rates, usually per thousand of the population at risk. Incidence rates are useful in tracking the rise and fall of the occurrence of a disease or a disorder and in seeking clues to its cause. Prevalence rates can be used to make inferences about incidence and cause as well as to plan services.

In epidemiological studies of mental retardation (MR), consideration of incidence is precluded by the wide variation in causal factors, which result in a range of characteristics; aside from some disorders known to be present at birth or the result of postnatal injury, researchers are unable to identify the onset. Thus, studies of MR in children or adults, by definition, yield prevalence rates.

The population at risk is limited to a geographically defined area, which may be a city, town, or rural area, or a region that encompasses urban and rural areas. Prevalence rates are most enlightening when the totals are broken down by severity of MR, age, sex, and a measure of socioeconomic status, such as social class. This information on the distribution of MR in the population can provide valuable insights into causally related factors and thus a basis for comparing studies at different times and places. It can also be used to make inferences about the effects of local conditions on the disorder and to judge whether the incidence may be increasing or decreasing over time. Because prevalence rates include all cases known to exist, mortality rates must be examined to determine if the frequency of new cases is actually changing or if variations in prevalence are due to changes in mortality.

Defining the Disorder

In any epidemiological inquiry, it is essential to identify those who do and do not have the disorder in question. Differences in definition will affect prevalence rates. There are several problems in definition particular to mental retardation, and these are reflected in the nine successive revisions of the definition made by the American Association on Mental Retardation (AAMR). The current definition, from the ninth edition of *Mental Retardation* (1992, p. 1), is based on the following three criteria:

1. *Subaverage intellectual functioning:* defined as a standardized measure of intelligence that gives an IQ of approximately 70 to 75 or below. The test must be appropriate to the individual's cultural, linguistic, and social background.
2. *Adaptive skill level:* limitations in adaptive skills must be documented within the context of community environments typical of the individual's age peers, and must exist in two or more of these areas: communication, self-care, home living, social skills, community use, self-direction, health and safety, functional academics, leisure, and work. A similar criterion is given by the World Health Organization: "Marked impairment in the ability of the individual to adapt to the daily demands of the social environment" (see WHO 1985, p. 8).
3. *Onset:* must be prior to age 18.

A person who meets these criteria has mental retardation at the time of the diagnosis, but it is not necessarily a permanent state: "Mental retardation disappears only when the individual is able to function well in the community without any additional supports or services beyond those provided to all citizens in the community (such as police and fire protection)" (AAMR 1992, p. 18).

A new element in the ninth edition is the recognition that the description of the individual's state of functioning must be viewed in the context of the structure and expectations of the individual's personal and social environments. The ninth edition also includes a statement about what mental retardation is *not:* it is not a medical or mental disorder, and it is not defined by particular etiological categories, although these may be variously present in persons with mental retardation.

The use of these diagnostic criteria makes identification of children with severe mental retardation relatively straightforward, except when severe sensory or motor disabilities complicate assessment. Problems arise most often in diagnosing a child whose IQ is toward the upper end of the IQ range for mental retardation. This difficulty is recognized in the AAMR definition, which gives an upper IQ limit of 70 to 75. The cut-off ranges in levels of adaptive behavior are not clearly defined and, even with detailed diagnostic assessments, considerable subjectivity in making decisions still remains possible.

Other Epidemiological Considerations

Time and place, as well as local conditions and circumstances, heavily influence epidemiologic studies. In planning and carrying out such studies, a number of considerations need to be taken into account, especially in studies of mild mental retardation.

Cultural Values and Social Factors

Until the 1950s or 1960s, segregation of children with MR in special classes, schools, or residential institutions had widespread acceptance. IQ testing was widely used for both administrative and research purposes. In the last quarter century, however, concern about the possible stigmatizing consequences of classifying a child as mentally retarded has been a growing, along with a recognition that segregating children with MR cuts them off from the social experiences important in preparing them for functioning as an adult in the society. As a consequence, the concept of "normalization" became influential, and, in some places, children with mild mental retardation were mainstreamed in regular classes. For fear of labeling and stigmatizing children, widespread IQ testing fell into disrepute, and researchers could no longer rely on the availability of IQ's to help identify children with mental retardation, or even routinely obtain relevant information from the educational authorities.

Fear of the stigma of mental retardation has had other consequences. In Scandinavia, it has been reported that psychologists have become more lenient in testing children, and this practice has led to higher scores, as discussed below. Teachers, once an important source of early identification of mental retardation because of their knowledge of the children in their classes, have become increasingly reluctant to assist in such identification. An increasing skepticism of the IQ test has also developed. As Mittler (1979) cautioned,

> Most psychologists are now well aware of the limitations of placing too much emphasis on an IQ score in judging the presence or extent of mental handicap. It is important to stress that the IQ is in no sense a "magic" number. Unfortunately, it has been credited with a degree of psychological significance out of all proportion either to its scientific status or its relevance to the practical problems of normal or handicapped persons. (p. 23)

These changes in professional values have increased the problems epidemiologists must face in identifying all children in the community with mental retardation.

Problems with IQ Tests

Tests of IQ vary, but all have a normal Gaussian distribution, with a mean score of 100 for the population on which it was standardized. They are not restandardized each time IQ testing is carried out on a new population. Continued use of the same test over time, without restandardization, has in fact been common practice. There is evidence, however, that over time children's performance has improved, and this has led to periodic revision. The Stanford-Binet was restandardized several times. In Sweden, when Sonnander (1990) administered the Wechsler Intelligence Scale for Children, standardized in the 1960s, on a representative school population, the mean score was 108, showing a clear upward drift. The greater the upward drift, the fewer the children there will be with IQ scores below 70 or 75. It is not clear whether children have become more intelligent or whether the upward drift is some artifact of the test. Flynn (1987) examined IQ trends around the world since 1950. Drawing on data from fourteen locations, mainly in Western Europe but also in Japan, the United States, Canada, New Zealand, and Australia, he showed IQ gains over one generation ranging from 5 to 25 points, with a median of 15, or a full standard deviation. Flynn concluded that "IQ tests do not really measure intelligence, but rather a correlate with a weak causal link to intelligence" (p. 190). Whatever the case may be, it poses a dilemma for those who use IQ testing as a component in identifying mental retardation and in the definition of mental retardation.

Census Data

To calculate a prevalence rate, in addition to obtaining the number of children in a particular age range with mental retardation (the numerator), it is also necessary to obtain the total number of children in the age range in the geographic area being studied (the denominator) from an age-specific census taken at the time the study is done. Further, if investigators wish to determine how children with MR are distributed in the population on characteristics such as social class, they must know how these characteristics distribute in the total population.

Adaptive Behavior

To meet the requirements of the current definition of mental retardation, the level of adaptive behavior must be considered along with intellectual level. To date, no attempt has been made to do systematic testing of adaptive behavior, using the available scales, in any community prevalence study. There have, however, been attempts to consider competence in skills now subsumed under the definition of adaptive behavior. The classroom and the broader school environment have always provided a good opportunity for teachers to assess performance in school work, and functioning on the playground, at lunch, sports, and other extracurricular activities. When concern about a child's adaptive behavior arose, the school authorities often consulted with the parents to obtain a second perspective. Even if a child had an IQ within the MR range, he or she would not necessarily be classified as MR if reasonable performance in school work and behavior was evident. Conversely, a child in the borderline area of IQ might have been classified as MR if he or she were unable to function adequately in regular classes and day-to-day life in school.

These issues are relevant largely to studies of mild mental retardation. For children with severe mental retardation, the evidence is generally apparent, and identification of all children with severe MR in a community does not present the same difficulties. For complete enumeration of these children, it is important to identify any children with severe MR from the population at risk who may have been sent out of the community for residential care.

Age

The more severe the mental retardation, the younger the age at which it will be identified. Severe MR is generally evident prior to school entry (unless it is caused by later insults or injuries). Children with mild MR are frequently not identified until the school years, when intellectual demands increase as the children grow older.

Most epidemiological studies have focused on children during the school years. Because the present study followed the children into young adulthood, it was possible to examine prevalence after school-leaving age. To do this, it is important to know how many children, identified as having mental retardation, continued to be so recognized and thus in need of adult MR services. Gruenberg (1964) reported on a number of studies in which the total prevalence dropped by approximately one half in the immediate postschool years.

The circumstances under which the present study was carried out were singularly propitious for identifying children with MR and obtaining relevant information on the population at risk. (See Chapter 2 for a description of these circumstances.)

Cumulative Prevalence

Prevalence: Total and by IQ

Our study population was defined as any child born between 1951 and 1955 and resident in Aberdeen in 1962 who had been administratively classified as MR at any time up to age 15. This resulted in complete ascertainment, yielding a cumulative prevalence of 16 per 1000, 3.3 per 1000 for severe MR and 12.7 per 1000 for mild MR. When the range of mild MR was subdivided by IQ, the prevalence rates for those with IQ 50–59, 60–69, and 70+ were, respectively, 3.5, 5.7, and 3.5 per 1000. Some studies use an upper cut-off point for mild MR of IQ 70. If we had adopted this cut-off point, the total prevalence would be 12.5 per 1000, with 9.2 per 1000 for children with IQ's of 50–69.

Gender

The ratios of boys with MR to girls with MR varied by IQ. In the mild MR IQ range of 50–69, the numbers of boys and girls were virtually the same. Among those with severe MR (IQ < 50), there was an excess of boys of 1.19:1.00, and among those with IQ 70+, there was an excess of boys of 2.2:1.00.

Social Class

Chapter 14 provides a full discussion of the social class measure, and the reasons for combining classes I–IIIa and breaking up social class III. As used here, social class I–IIIa represents nonmanual work, and social class V represents unskilled manual labor. The concept of social class has been widely used in epidemiological studies to provide a broad indicator of family life styles. The prevalence by social class is shown for the four IQ categories (see Figure 5.1). Eighteen children were excluded because they could not be assigned a social class. For those with IQ <50, the prevalence by social class appears random, but highest for social class V. The skewing of the distribution toward higher prevalence at the lower end of the social class scale is most marked for the children with IQ 60–69, where there is a stepwise increase from upper to lower social class. The skewing is present but less marked for those with IQ of 70+, and it is even less clear for IQ 50–59. For the IQ categories of 60–69 and 70+, the prevalence of social class V is greater than for all other social classes combined.

In each social class and IQ category, we wanted to determine whether the numbers were more or less than would be expected by chance alone. To determine the expected number, we used the following calculation: (total number at risk of MR in the social class)

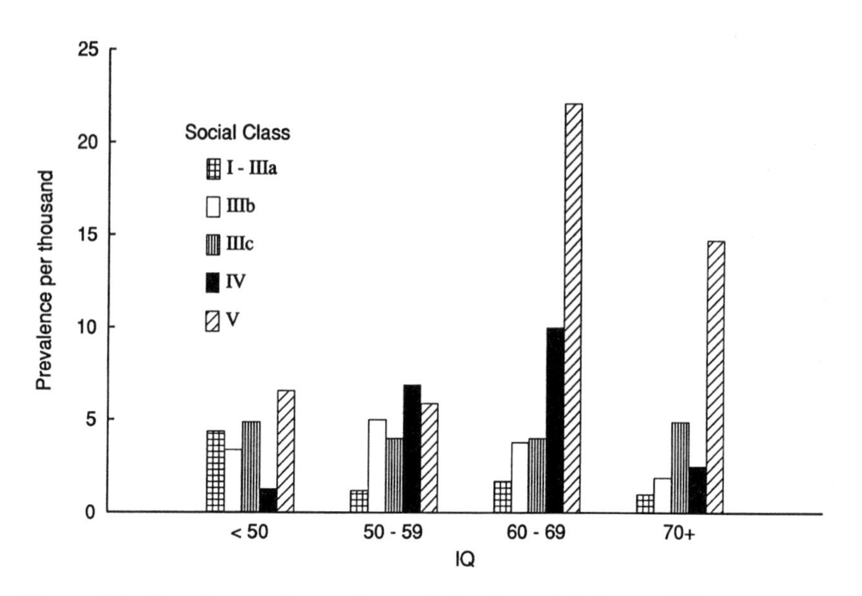

Figure 5.1 Prevalence of mental retardation by social class and IQ group.

× (total number of children in the social class who had MR) ÷ (the total of children in all social classes). If dividing the *expected* number by the *actual* number in a social class yields a result that is greater than 1, there is overrepresentation in that social class, and if it is less than 1, there is underrepresentation. The results are shown in Figure 5.2. In social classes I–IIIa, children with IQ below 50 were overrepresented, but throughout the mild MR range, they were underrepresented. The largest overrepresentation in the mild MR range occurred for children in social classes IV and V with IQ's of 60–69.

We were unable to assign a social class for eighteen children, because they had experienced unstable caretaker histories during their upbringing—some had lived in hostels for children and some had been fostered with more than one family—or because they had been raised in families where neither parent had had a sufficient job history that would allow a classification of their occupation. No prevalence by social class could be calculated for these children, since we had no way of ascertaining the denominator data—the total number of children in the community for whom it was impossible to assign a social class. It is reasonable to postulate that conditions for most of these children during their upbringing were unfavorable for effective socialization, and that their characteristics would be more akin to children at the lower than at the upper end of the social class scale.

Because we could not obtain a prevalence rate for these children, we used other methods for comparative purposes. Figure 5.3 shows how IQ is distributed within each social class and among those who were not classifiable. Among those not classifiable (NC), the IQ distribution was closest to that in social class V. At each step down the social class scale, the percentage with IQ's of 60 and above increased; this stepwise increase extended to the unclassified children, who had the largest percentage with IQ's of 60 and above. Conversely, for the children with IQ <50, the progression was in the opposite direction, although without as clear a gradient as for those with IQ 60 and above. In social class I–IIIa, 50 percent had IQ <50, almost twice the proportion in any other social class.

Age-Specific Prevalence

Age-specific prevalence rates provide information for estimating service needs at different stages of life. They also provide better infor-

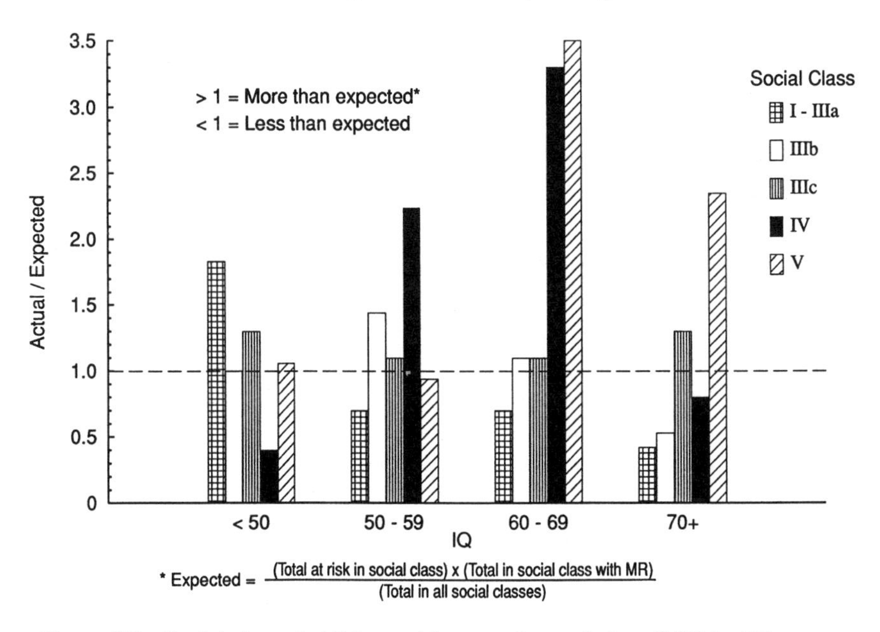

Figure 5.2 Social class of children with mental retardation (MR) by IQ group, shown as actual versus expected numbers.

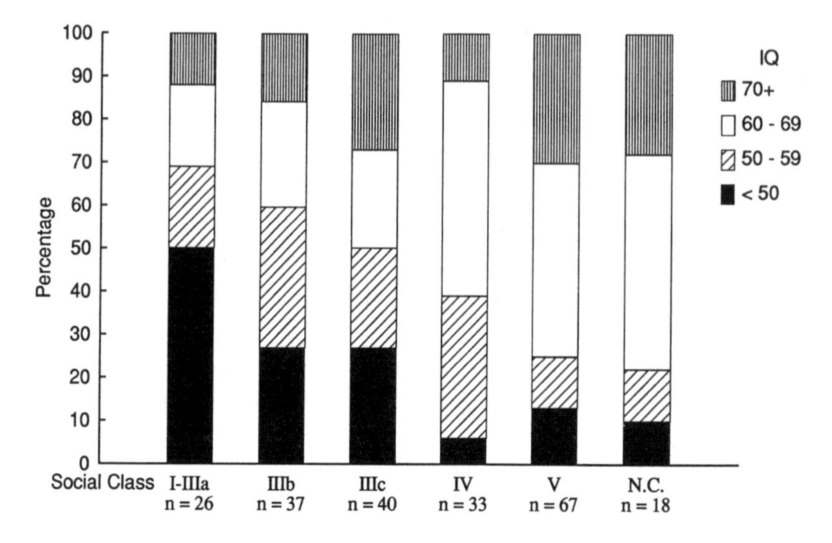

Figure 5.3 Percentages of children with mental retardation by IQ group and social class, including those not classifiable (NC).

mation for making comparisons with other prevalence studies of mental retardation, which are, for the most part, reported for specified age ranges. Because we knew the ages at which the children in our study were classified as MR and followed them to age 22, we were able to examine age-specific prevalence rates. Prevalence rates increased as new children were identified, and they decreased because of deaths, transfers back to regular classes, and disappearance from MR services after leaving school. This last reason for a drop in prevalence at school-leaving is widespread across communities. During the school years, compulsory education makes age-specific demands on children to meet minimum standards of school performance and behavior. After they leave school, the demands made on young adults are far more flexible, because the tasks and roles expected of them offer a much wider set of options. In school, the demands of literacy, numeracy, and language usage are primary. In some jobs, however, such as unskilled manual labor, these are less important. Although some young adults classified as mentally retarded during the school years might be able to function in the postschool world without the need for adult MR services, others require these services for some or all of their adult lives.

The age-specific administrative prevalence rates from ages 5 to 22 for the total population classified as MR reflect these considerations (see Figure 5.4). Beginning at age 5, the prevalence increased annually, reaching a plateau at ages 11 and 12, and then showed a slight annual decline until school-leaving at ages 15 to 16. Following the school years, between ages 14 and 16, the prevalence dropped by slightly over a half; after age 16 it showed some small annual decline. At no age was the prevalence as high as the cumulative prevalence of 16 per 1000. The progression of age-specific prevalence was similar to that demonstrated by Gruenberg in 1964.

Most children were classified as MR by age 8, but some not until age 13. Between ages 8 and 14, nineteen children improved sufficiently in their school functioning to warrant their return to regular classes. There was also some reduction in prevalence because of six deaths between ages 6 and 13, and four deaths between ages 16 and 22. The remainder of the reduction was the result of the disappearance of almost half the young people from MR services after school-leaving age. Whether they continued to function poorly as young adults, or whether their adjustment and quality of life made them indistinguishable from nonretarded peers with similar backgrounds,

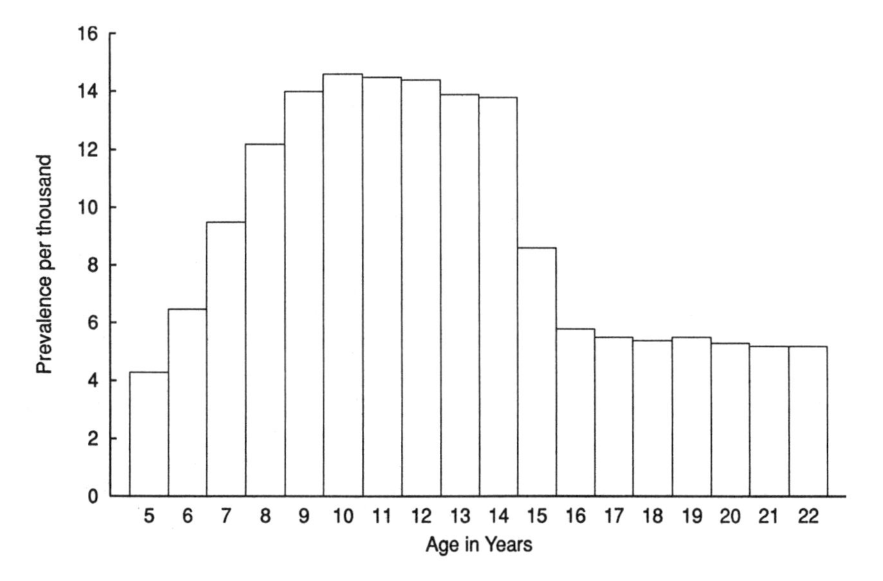

Figure 5.4 Age-specific prevalence of mental retardation.

is one of the central issues of the study, and will be addressed in later chapters.

Severity of Mental Retardation

The patterns of age-specific prevalence differed, depending on the degree of severity of the MR (see Figure 5.5). For those with severe MR (IQ <50), the peak prevalence occurred at an early age and showed a slight decline thereafter due almost entirely to deaths.

Those with IQ 60–69 showed the steepest rise and fall of prevalence with age; as the largest of the IQ groups, they also contributed most to the overall changes in prevalence. The IQ groups of 50–59 and 70+ likewise contributed to the rise and fall in prevalence but to a lesser degree. Among the population with IQ 50+, the decline in prevalence was due in part to the fact that some children returned to regular schools but more generally to their disappearance from MR services after leaving school. There were two deaths among those with IQ 70+ at age 18, one a known, and the other a suspected, suicide. The sharpest drop in prevalence after school leaving was found for those with IQ 70+, which is not surprising.

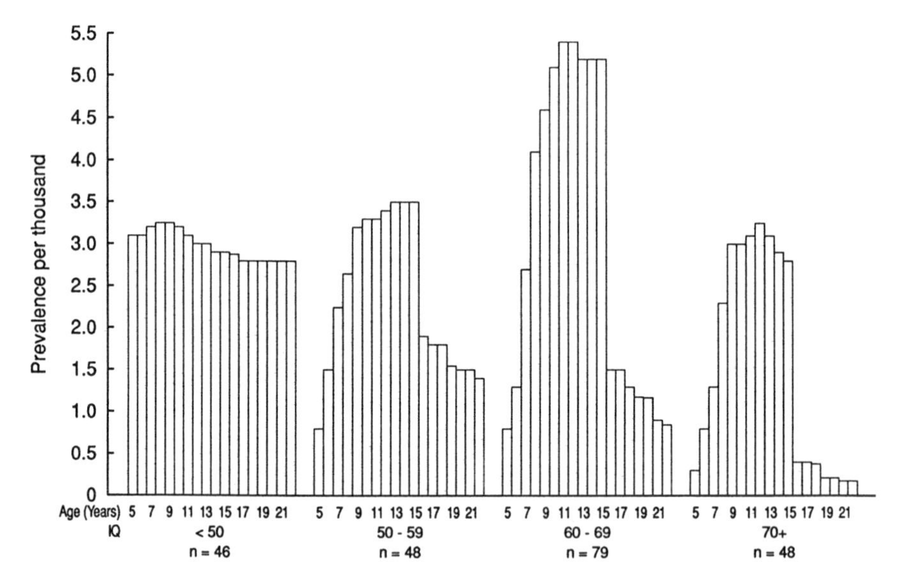

Figure 5.5 Age-specific prevalence of mental retardation by IQ group.

Gender

Figure 5.6 shows the ratio of males to females by age. The largest excess of males was found at age 5 and dropped rapidly at ages 6 and 7. The high ratio of boys to girls at age 5 was found at all IQ levels. From age 7, when the sex ratio was 1.11:1.00, the trend was an increasing boy/girl ratio until age 16. After age 18, there was almost no excess of males.

Social Class

Figure 5.7 shows the prevalence rates by social class for selected ages: the lower the social class, the greater the increase in prevalence between ages 7 and 11. For this age period, the prevalence rates doubled in social classes IV and V but nowhere else. The increases with age occurred most markedly for those with IQ's of 60 and above. After school-leaving, the drop in prevalence shown for age 19 was greatest for social classes IV and V; within these classes, it was greatest for young people with IQ's of 60–69 and even more so for those with IQ's of 70+. As these results make clear, when prevalence rates by social class are compared across studies, the ages of the populations being compared need to be taken into account.

We were unable to obtain prevalence rates for children who could not be assigned a social class. Using numbers rather than prevalence

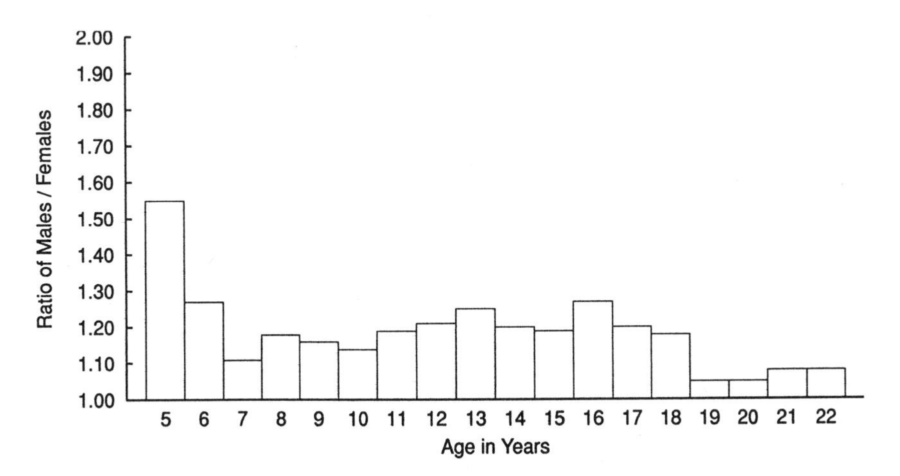

Figure 5.6 Ratios of males to females with mental retardation by age.

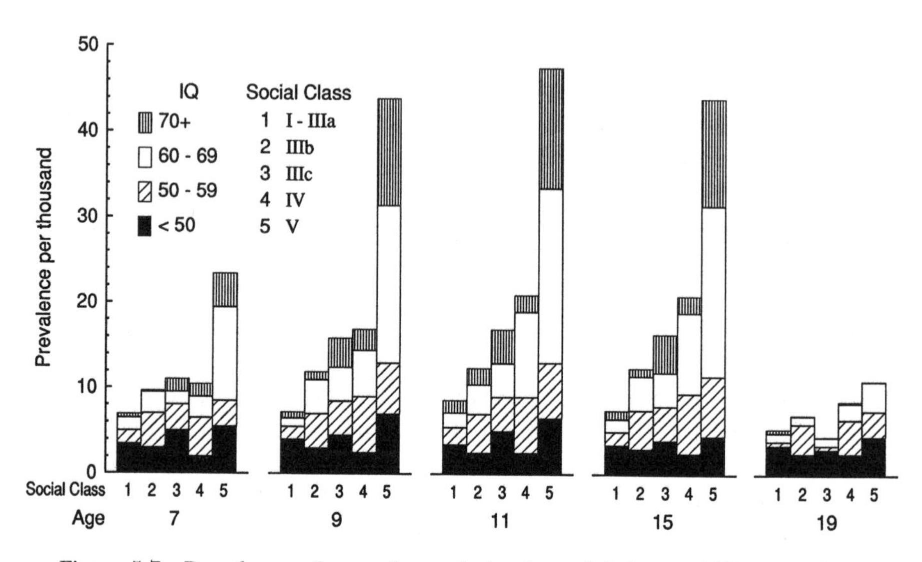

Figure 5.7 Prevalence of mental retardation by social class and IQ group for selected ages.

rates, Figure 5.8 shows that higher percentages of the children who were not classifiable were placed in the special school at earlier ages than children in social classes IV and V.

Services

Age-specific prevalence rates for the various types of services are of value in planning MR services. In the United States at the time of our study, the primary concern about services for people with MR was deinstitutionalization and the organization of group homes. These services were essential because of a heritage of large-scale institutional placement. What has been learned from this experience, however, will have little relevance for the future, when children with MR will be kept whenever possible within a family setting or elsewhere in the community.

Between 1956 and 1972, the present study population was of school age and between 1967 and 1977, aged 17 to 22. Although some changes in patterns of services have occurred since that time, the rates may be useful as estimates of the kinds of service needs in a total representative population of young people with MR.

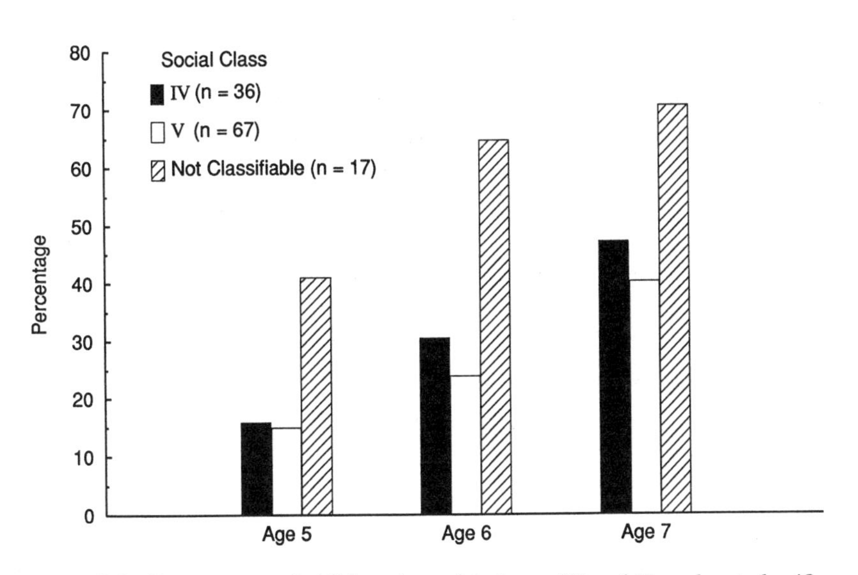

Figure 5.8 Percentages of children in social classes IV and V, and not classifiable (NC), who were in mental retardation services at ages 5, 6, and 7.

Chapter 15, which deals with the study population's experiences with MR services, provides a longitudinal perspective of individual paths through services. Here, we give the prevalence rates for the various MR services and briefly describe each one.

Children's Services

Special school. The special school served children who were too intellectually limited to cope in regular classes but were expected to benefit from small classes with specially trained teachers.

Junior Occupation Center (JOC). The JOC served children with more severe MR, who were unable to benefit from the program at the special school.

Residential care. There were several forms of residential care for children with MR. In order to calculate prevalence rates, we will combine them here (in Chapter 15 they are considered separately).

A few children, all with severe MR, remained at home during the day and were cared for by their parents, with some assistance from the health and educational authorities.

Adult Services

Senior Occupational Centers (SOC's). Several SOC's provided day programs for the young people who were unable to cope in open employment and lived in the community with their parents or parent substitutes. The programs offered social training, and some included vocational training and recreational facilities. At one of the centers, there were facilities for caring for adults with severe and multiple disabilities.

Residential care. Several residential facilities served adults who were from Aberdeen. For calculating prevalence, they were combined.

Prevalence Rates in Childhood

The age-specific prevalence rates for the various forms of services are shown in Figure 5.9. The childhood years from ages 6 to 16 are shown for the special school and the JOC, and the postschool years from 16 to 22 for the SOC's. Residential placements spanned the years from childhood through to age 22, and home care to age 18. During the school years, by far the largest number of children were in the special school, and the numbers increased rapidly, from a prevalence of 2.5

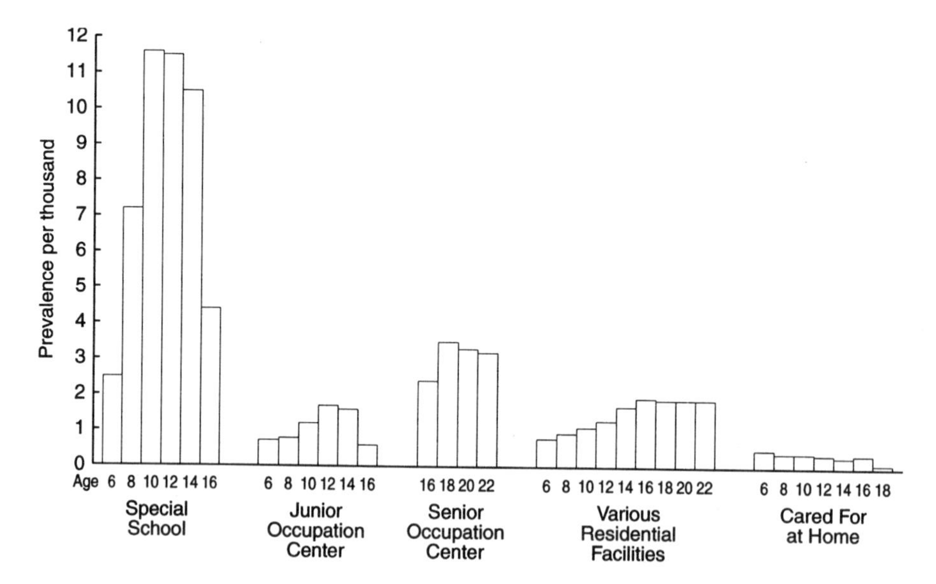

Figure 5.9 Prevalence in various mental retardation services by age.

per 1000 at age 6 to 11.8 per 1000 by age 10. At age 14 the prevalence dropped to 10.2 because some children returned to regular schools and some were transferred to various residential facilities. The precipitous drop in prevalence between 15 and 17 years of age was due to leaving school over this two-year period.

The prevalence rate per 1000 children at the JOC was 0.7 at age 6 and increased to 1.8 at age 15, before dropping sharply during the school-leaving period.

The rates for residential care are shown for the whole age range from 6 to 22. They revealed a slight steady rise, from 0.8 per 1000 at age 6 to 1.9 per 1000 at age 16, where they reached a plateau.

The least frequent form of service in childhood was that provided by parents who kept their children at home. There was a decrease in prevalence with age because of some deaths and some transfers to other forms of service.

Prevalence in the Postschool Years

For the postschool years, the prevalence of people in day services was nearly twice the rate of those in residential services. The age-specific rates in day services increased from 2.4 to 3.5 per 1000 in the first two years after school-leaving because some young people were transferred directly from the JOC, and some who tried employment initially were unable to cope. After age 18, the prevalence remained relatively constant.

The number of young people between ages 17 and 22 in residential care remained almost unchanged. Except for one who died, those who had been cared for at home during childhood had all been moved into an adult day service by age 20.

The prevalence rates given are cross-sectional by age and are useful as estimates for planning services. The rates have not been subdivided by gender, IQ, or type of residential care. In Chapter 15, we will describe the career paths of the young people across the two periods of childhood and young adulthood, and examine IQ, disabilities, gender, and type of residential care in some detail.

Children Who Met Only the Psychometric Criterion for Mental Retardation

As we have noted, the current definition of mental retardation (AAMR 1992) requires that, along with being identified as having

MR in childhood, individuals must meet two additional criteria. Children meeting the psychometric but not the adaptive behavior criterion do not fit the current definition. Rutter et al. (1970b) used the term "intellectual retardation" to describe these children. Not all investigators are that precise, however, and many prevalence studies have been carried out using only a psychometric definition.

We found it possible to calculate prevalence rates for children who remained in regular classes throughout their schooling but scored below 75 on group intelligence tests because these tests were administered to every child in Aberdeen at ages 7 and 9. Based on the results of the age 9 test, the prevalence of IQ <75 in regular classes was 13.3 per 1000. If this were added to the 14 per 1000 children classified (see Figure 5.4), this yields a prevalence of approximately 27 percent, a rate close to the theoretical prevalence based on the Gaussian curve of IQ. Figure 5.10 shows the social class distribution of these children and of the children with IQ's of 60 and greater who had been administratively classified as MR. (This is similar to the range of IQ's of the psychometrically defined group in regular classes.) The two distributions are similar, indicating that these children

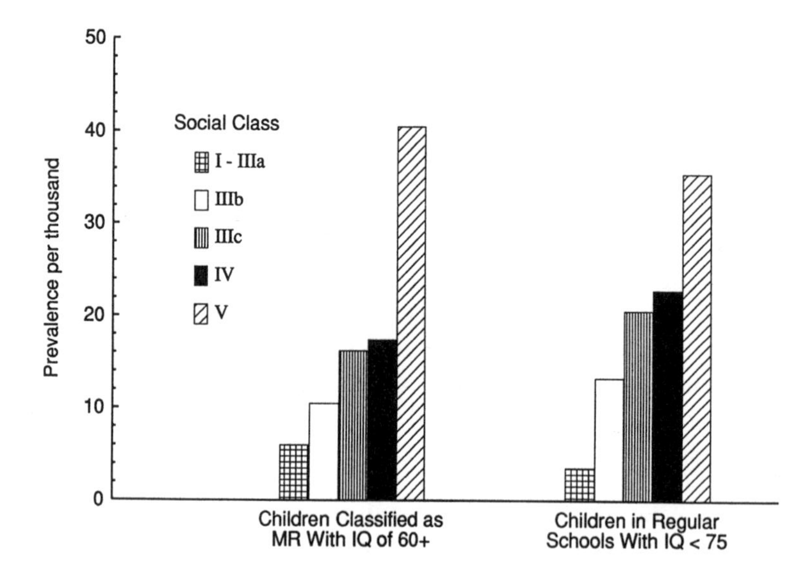

Figure 5.10 Social class prevalence of children with similar IQ's who were and were not classified as mentally retarded (MR) at age 9.

came from similar social backgrounds and that there was no social class bias in the selection for special school placement.

Comparison of Results with Other Studies

As Fryers (1987) has pointed out, definitions of severe mental retardation and mild mental retardation involve separate considerations.

> IQ alone has not usually been considered sufficient for defining "retardation" (Clarke and Clarke 1985), but all people with an IQ below 50, at all ages, in all societies and in all services will be considered retarded, and no other feature is *necessary* for this category. Therefore, IQ is actually the sole criterion for definition and "Severe Mental Retardation/ Handicap" is co-terminus with "Severe Intellectual Impairment." This is clearly not so for milder degrees of intellectual impairment and there is, therefore, a conceptual discontinuity between severe and mild MR. (p. 368)

For mild MR it is necessary to take into account adaptive behavior, the second criterion in the definition of mental retardation. Mittler (1979) noted that "it is obvious that many people with IQ's lower than 70 manage reasonably well and do not require special help" (p. 28).

From these considerations, it seems clear that the prevalence rate for severe MR obtained in the follow-up study may reasonably be compared to studies based only on a psychometric definition. However, to obtain a meaningful prevalence rate for mild MR, it is necessary to use, in addition to a psychometric definition, some criteria that are indicative of adaptive behavior.

Severe Mental Retardation

Prevalence studies of MR have largely dealt with severe MR, and there are numerous reviews (Richardson and Koller 1994; Abramowicz and Richardson 1975; Akesson 1986; Fryers 1984, 1987, 1991, 1992; Gruenberg 1964; Kiely 1987; Kushlick and Blunden 1974; Lapouse and Weitzner 1970; McLaren and Bryson 1987; Munro 1986). They indicate that the prevalence of severe MR ranges from approximately

2 per 1000 to 7 per 1000. Since these reviews, Murphy et al. (1995), in a study of 10-year-old children in Atlanta, Georgia, found a prevalence rate of 3.6 per 1000. In our follow-up study, the cumulative prevalence of severe MR was 3.3 per 1000. The age-specific prevalence ranged from 3.3 per 1000 at ages 8 and 9 to 2.8 per 1000 at age 22, the drop due almost exclusively to mortality. Our prevalence, then, is within the range of other studies and close to the median prevalence for children of 3.7 per 1000 suggested by Abramowicz and Richardson (1975) and the rate given by Murphy et al. The present study is also in accord with previous studies in showing a slight excess of males of 1.19:1.00.

Most previous studies of severe MR have shown that prevalence is random across the social classes. A few have found the highest prevalence at the low end of the social class scale. Our results also show a random distribution across social class, with the highest prevalence at the low end (social class V).

The number of children testing around the upper cut-off point for severe MR of IQ 50 may differ. A relatively small shift in numbers of children immediately above and below the cut-off point will affect the prevalence.

Research on successive birth cohorts of children studied in the same place (Fryers 1984; Martindale et al. 1988), has demonstrated that there are secular trends in the age-specific prevalence of severe MR, but these have not shown a consistent steady increase or decrease over a long period of time.

Mild Mental Retardation

In addition to the IQ criterion for mental retardation, the present study used the judgment of the educational authorities that the child did not meet the minimal age-specific expectations for school performance and behavior.

Our results have shown how prevalence varied, depending on whether the rate was cumulative or age-specific, what IQ cut-off point was used, and whether only IQ or, in addition, an administrative classification was used. Table 5.1 shows how prevalence rates varied in our study, depending on age and on the definition of mild MR used. During childhood, prevalence rates ranged from 5 per 1000 to 26 per 1000, made up of all children classified with IQ's of 50+ and

Table 5.1 Prevalence rates of mild MR in our follow-up study using different definitions

Definition of MR	Rate
A. *Cumulative Prevalence*	
Psychometric definitions of mild MR	
Children administratively classified as MR, with IQ 50 and above (12.7/1000), and children in regular classes with IQ below 75 (13.3/1000)	26.0/1000
Administratively classified as MR	
IQ 50 and above	12.7/1000
IQ 50–69	9.4/1000
B. *Age-Specific Prevalence*	
Administratively classified as MR	
Age 12, with IQ 50 and above	11.8/1000
Age 12, with IQ 50–69	8.8/1000
Age 7, with IQ 50 and above	6.3/1000
Age 7, with IQ 50–69	5.0/1000
Age 22, with IQ 50 and above	2.5/1000
Age 22, with IQ 50–69	2.3/1000

children with IQ's <75 in regular classes. By age 22, only 2.3 per 1000 to 2.5 per 1000 remained classified as MR because they were still receiving services.

In comparing our results with previous research, we were able to conform to the various definitions of MR used in other studies. We found five prevalence studies that used the two criteria of IQ and placement in special schools (Table 5.2). For all but the Stein et al. (1976) study, the prevalence rates were given by the authors. For this exception we calculated the prevalence from the data they presented. Stein et al. (1976) obtained scores on the Raven's Progressive Matrices from military records for 19-year-old survivors of all males born 1944–1947, a period that included the Dutch famine of 1944–1945. These data were unique in that they were national and virtually total for the whole population of more than 400,000 males. Scores with IQ equivalents of 50–55 up to about 75 were used to define mild MR. This gave a psychometric prevalence rate of 57.6 per 1000. Stein et al. reported that 30.5 per 1000 of the study population had attended special schools, and 57 percent of these individuals had also met the psychometric criterion of mild MR, resulting in a prevalence of 17.4

Table 5.2 Studies of mild MR that have used the two criteria of IQ and educational classification

Reference	Place	Definition of mild MR	Ages	Prevalence per 1000	Present study per 1000[a]
Drillien, Jameson, and Wilkinson 1966	Edinburgh, Scotland	Children considered unsuited for education in ordinary classes because of mental subnormality with IQ 50–69	7–14	6.3	7.9
Sorel 1974	Amsterdam, Holland	Registered as mentally retarded with IQ 50–69	13	9.6	8.7
Stein, Susser, and Saenger 1976	Netherlands	Previous attendance at special school and IQ equivalent of Raven's Progressive Matrices of 50–75, males only	19	17.4	13.9
Murphy et al. 1995	Atlanta, Georgia	Children administratively classified and placed in special facilities for MR, IQ 50–69	10	8.4	8.5

a. Calculated for the age, IQ range, and sex of the study being compared.

per 1000. This rate was based on the assumption that the scores on the Raven's test accurately reflected IQ's in childhood. No permanent effects of the Dutch famine during World War II in reducing intellectual functioning were found, but it is possible that the prevalence rate in this study was influenced by that event.

It is noteworthy that four of these studies were published in the 1960s and 1970s, and the remaining one in 1995, and that they were carried out in four different countries. Despite these differences in time and place, our prevalence rates were very close to theirs when we used similar definitions.

A number of studies have been carried out using only a psychometric criterion of mild MR, with an IQ range of 50–69 (Table 5.3), but again, they were conducted when no restrictions were placed on widespread intelligence testing. The Lemkau and Imre (1968) study yielded prevalence rates three to four times higher than the others.

A probable explanation is that the study dealt primarily with rural children of low social class. In our follow-up study, prevalence rates were far higher in the lower than in the upper social classes. The Gruenberg (1955) prevalence is the lowest, probably because IQ data for nearly half of the children were unavailable. The three remaining

Table 5.3 Prevalence of MR based on psychometric criteria only and under conditions where large-scale testing of children was acceptable

Reference	Place	Description of study	Ages	Prevalence per 1000
Rutter, Tizard, and Whitmore 1970	Isle of Wight	Initial multiple testing to screen children. Then IQ testing on those scoring low on screening. Definition of MR: all children with IQ ≥ 2 standard deviations below Mean IQ for all children on the island.	8–10	22.3[a]
Lemkau and Imre 1968	Southeast U.S., rural low-income population	All children screened on various tests. Those with lower scores given IQ tests.	6–9 10–14	66 89
Gruenberg 1955	Onondaga County, New York	Child identified by child-care agencies with possible or certain MR. Estimated prevalence based on children for whom IQ tests were available with scores of 75 and below.	5–17	18.3
Granat and Granat 1973	Sweden	Sample of Swedish inductees for compulsory medical service. Those with est. IQ <70 based on six tests from Ulleracker Sjukhus battery of tests and those already classified as MR.	19	22.1
Birch et al. 1970	Aberdeen, Scotland	All children born 1952–54 resident in Aberdeen in 1962 who were classified as MR and all children in regular classes with IQ <75 on a group IQ test.	8–10	27.4

a. When the norms given in the test instructions were used, the prevalence was 15.5.

studies give a range of prevalence rates of 22 per 1000 to 27 per 1000, which is very close to the approximately 25 per 1000 expected from the theoretical Gaussian distribution of intelligence tests. Because of the general pattern of upward drift in test performance, the psychometric prevalence based on tests that have not recently been restandardized would be lower. When Rutter et al. (1970b) restandardized test norms to define intellectual retardation, the prevalence rate dropped from 22.3 per 1000 to 15.5 per 1000.

Some prevalence studies of mild MR have been based on health registers, but these only include children with health problems or disabilities. While this would encompass almost all children with severe MR, because severe MR is strongly related to other disabilities, the same is not true for mild MR. As Table 5.4 shows, the prevalence rates for mild MR based on health registers are far lower than prevalence rates based on school classification.

In a series of studies of the prevalence of mild MR among Swedish children published in the 1980s, rates ranged from 3.6 per 1000 to 5.6 per 1000 (see Table 5.5). These low rates elicited considerable international attention. Gallagher (1985) summarized the way these results were interpreted in Sweden: "They are maximizing variables in this

Table 5.4 Prevalence of mild MR on the basis of health registers

Reference	Place	Definition	Age	Prevalence per 1000
Bayley 1973	Sheffield, England	"Subnormals on the books of the Sheffields Mental Health Services," 1968	5–9 10–14 15–19	0.06 0.46 0.78
Kushlick and Blunden 1974	Salford, England	Salford register of mentally deficient persons kept by local health authority, 1961	5–9 10–14 15–19	0.36 0.29 8.63
Kushlick and Blunden 1974	Wessex, England	Mental defectives known to Mental Health Depts. of local health authorities, psychiatric hospitals, and private residences	5–9 10–14 15–19	0.57 0.48 2.97
Wallner 1988	Sweden[a]	Children registered with Board of Provisions and Services of Mentally Retarded Persons	5–9 10–14 15–19	0.8 3.1 4.0

a. Mild MR prevalence based on total prevalence minus 3.3/1000 estimated severe MR.

multivariate formulation of adult-child linguistic interaction, subcultural family factors, and physical health conditions, and have minimized significant infant pathology through good prenatal and postnatal care" (p. 106). But this interpretation presumes that the prevalence rates were valid estimates of mild MR, a presumption that requires examination. The investigators defined mild MR solely on the basis of an IQ of 50 to 69. In Sweden, however, the IQ test had fallen into disrepute because it was feared that a low score would stigmatize a child. Under these conditions, the investigators were unable to administer intelligence tests. Only some of the children with IQ 50–69 were identified as having mild MR and enrolled in special classes. Unknown numbers of children in regular classes, who were not administratively defined as MR, must also have had IQ's below 70.

The children known to have MR were those registered with the Board for Provisions and Services to the Mentally Retarded (BPSMR). The usual requirements for enrollment were a medical certificate plus a psychological, pedagogical, and social investigation of the case (Wallner 1988). National prevalence rates, based on the register, were 4.1 per 1000 for ages 5 to 9, 6.4 per 1000 for 10 to 14 and 7.3 per 1000 for 15 to 19 (Wallner 1988). Sonnander (1990) has demonstrated that there had been an upward drift in intelligence test performance. For a total unselected, representative population of children in a large Swedish town, she obtained a mean IQ of 108. Gillberg et al. (1983) point to changing practices among psychologists: "These days, with more negative attitudes towards IQ testing among many psychologists, a 'wrong' answer is often interpreted positively and a 'try again' answer allowed" (p. 217). Under these difficult circumstances, investigators attempted to find children with IQ 50–69 who were not known to the BPSMR by asking for nominations from school nurses and psychologists or by screening the population with tests measuring intelligence only indirectly. From other studies that used a psychometric definition of mild MR, the prevalence, allowing for upward drift, probably should be around 15 per 1000, three to four times the prevalence rate found in Sweden.

It appears, then, that the Swedish studies found such low psychometrically defined prevalence rates of mild MR because investigators were unable to carry out widespread testing in a system where children with mild MR were often mainstreamed and thus remained unidentified. The children who were identified were mainly those with

Table 5.5 Prevalence of mild MR found in Scandinavian studies in the 1980s

Reference	Definition and Place	Method	Age	Prevalence per 1000	Notes
Hagberg et al. 1981a,b	Gothenberg, Sweden. IQ 50–70.	Terman Merrill or Wise Register (BPSMR)[a] and hospital children suspected by school nurses and psychologists.	8–12; born 1966–70	3.7	72 children in special, 19 in ordinary schools
Blomquist et al. 1981	Västerbotten County, N. Sweden: IQ 50–69 once registered with BPSMR.	IQ based on available records and interviews with teachers and school nurses.	8–15; born 1963–70	3.6	
Gillberg et al. 1983	Gothenberg, Sweden. IQ 50–70; WISC, 4th Swedish revised version.	BPSMR register search and screening 72% of population to detect perceptual, conceptual, motor, and attentional deficits. Screened children tested on Performance part of WISC. Tested age 8.	6–7; born 1971	5.6	23 found in BPsevere MR register; 28 not in register

(continued on p. 91)

various developmental disabilities in addition to IQ 50–69, and those with IQ's at the lower end of that range.

In all the studies of mild MR cited in this chapter, the prevalence increased as social class decreased. Further, there was a stepwise social class increase in the administrative prevalence of mild MR with age, the slope becoming steeper as age increased, because the children who were classified at older ages, generally with IQ's at the upper end of the mild MR range, were those most likely to come from lower

Table 5.5 (continued)

Reference	Definition and Place	Method	Age	Prevalence per 1000	Notes
Gostason 1985	Kopparberg County, Central Sweden. Swedish test SPIQ(159); Vocab. subtest (Swedish) revised Stanford Binet; IQ ≤73.7 and Stanford Binet ≤53.	BPSMR register. Children repeated a year in remedial classes; school records; various adult sources, including military records.	Adults 20–29.	5.3	
Kaariainen, Piepponen, and Vaskilampi 1985	Kupio Province, Finland. IQ 56–70.	Population screened with school achievement tests of reading and arithmetic. If those tested suggested MR, individual tests of verbal ability, visual perception.	8–9; born 1969–70, 1971–72.	4.1 11.3	
Rantakallio and von Wendt 1986	Finland; two most northerly provinces: Oulu and Lapland. Available IQ tests. Estimated Terman Merrill or WISC. IQ 50–70.	96% of children born in 1966. Followed up 1966–83.	Up to age 14.	5.5	

a. BPSMR—Board for Provisions and Service to the Mentally Retarded.

social class families. In comparing social class distributions across studies, it is necessary, then, to take account of the ages for which administrative prevalence is obtained and whether age-specific or cumulative prevalence is used. In studies that use a psychometric definition of mild MR, if all children are tested, then the distribution of social class prevalence is unlikely to change with age, assuming no drift in IQ's over time.

At different times and places, the social class distribution of a defined population will vary. We have shown that the psychometric prevalence of mild MR in a poor rural area (Lemkau and Imre 1968) was far higher than that in the other studies in Table 5.3, where there was not a predominance of low social class families.

For 8 percent of the present study population, it was not possible to assign a social class. In some cases, there was no head of household with a job history. The father, for example, had been chronically unemployed or had been disabled since before the child was born, and the family was supported by social security payments. In other cases, children were brought up in various forms of care, including hostels run by the local authorities, and a series of foster homes. Although it is likely that in other studies examining the social class of children with MR some had similar atypical histories, they are not mentioned. They may have been added to the numbers in the lowest social class. Because we had complete histories for the children in our follow-up study but were unable to assign a social class to some of them, we developed a measure of family stability, which encompassed these children (see Chapter 14).

Sex Differences

Our study is in accord with others in finding that, for total populations of children with MR, boys outnumber girls. For severe MR, results of previous studies have a median male/female ratio of between 1.2 and 1.3:1.00. The present study, with 1.21:1.00, fits within this range.

A review of sex differences in children administratively classified as having mild MR (Richardson et al. 1986b) concluded that boys almost always outnumbered girls and found the highest boy/girl ratio at the upper end of the IQ range used. The present study agreed, finding a boy/girl ratio of 1.22:1.00 for all those with IQ's of 50 and above, but the excess of boys was accounted for completely by those with IQ's of 70+; in this group, the boy/girl ratio was 2.2:1.00.

In two studies of children defined as having mild MR, where sex ratios were given at each year of age from 7 to 15 (Levinson 1962; Ramer 1946), the ratios of males to females showed a fairly steady increase with age (Richardson et al. 1986b). The follow-up study revealed a similar trend. A number of biomedical and cultural-familial factors may account for these sex differences. Among genetic factors, because boys have a single X chromosome, they are more vulnerable to the expression of a variety of disorders than girls, who have two X chromosomes. There are also specific X-linked disorders related to MR, the most common of which is the fragile-X syndrome, which affect more males than females, although the degree to which this occurs is still uncertain.

Several factors in the socialization of children may help explain why more boys are unable to meet the minimum standards for school performance and behavior than girls and, with IQ's at the upper end of the mild MR range, are thus classified as MR. Parents have had higher aspirations for sons, more than for daughters, both academically and vocationally. This has put more pressure on boys to succeed in school. "In kindergarten through the fourth grade," however, "the girl typically outperforms the boy in all areas, and the ratio of boys to girls with reading problems ranges from three-to-one to six-to-one" (Kagan 1964, p. 158). Girls at this stage tend to be taller than boys and more fluent verbally. Despite these differences, children are grouped in classes according to chronological age, which places boys at a disadvantage. This may increase the pressures on boys, especially if they have some intellectual limitations. (For a fuller account of factors leading to differences in the school performance of boys and girls, see Richardson et al. 1986a.)

Rutter et al. (1970b) summarized the biosocial interaction of these factors: "it has been suggested that the biological immaturity of the male leads to greater susceptibility to 'stress' of all kinds and that the reading retardation constitutes a stress response resulting from an interaction between physically based immaturity and the social and psychological demands on the child" (p. 46). To the extent that the socialization of girls is becoming more career- and achievement-oriented, it will be interesting to see whether this will lead to changes in the sex ratios of boys and girls with mild MR.

Cultures differ in the extent to which they treat boys and girls differently. This is suggested in a study of the prevalence of mental retardation in Kurume City, Japan. Shiotsuki et al. (1984) show a mean male/female ratio of 3.4:1.0 for children aged 7 to 12, a far higher ratio than found in any European studies, which may reflect cultural differences, despite the biological explanation the Japanese authors suggest.

Consequences of Normalization and Mainstreaming

The studies we have reviewed suggest that while in the 1970s and earlier some children with similar intellectual limitations would have been classified as mildly MR and placed in special classes, they now remain in regular classes and are not classified. The shift away from IQ testing and segregation into special classes and toward normalization and mainstreaming was based on the fear that labeling and special placement would be stigmatizing. Few considered that leaving children with intellectual limitations in regular classes might disadvantage and stigmatize them in other ways. The extent to which children with mild MR are stigmatized by being mainstreamed is likely to depend on the quality of the teaching and the size of the classes. In small classes taught by a competent teacher, the needs of children with a wide range of abilities, including mild MR, can be met; in large classes with less competent teachers, children with mild MR are likely to be stigmatized in their peer relationships and disadvantaged in their educational experiences. We need more research on children with mild MR who are not "labeled" and remain in regular classes to determine the nature of their school experiences and the extent to which they encounter problems and experience stigma.

Postschool Years

We examined age-specific administrative prevalence rates up to age 22, and the large drop after school-leaving age confirmed Gruenberg's (1964) conclusion: after leaving school, only the young adults who continued to receive mental retardation services, whether day or residential, were included in prevalence rates. About half of those administratively classified as MR during childhood continued as adults in MR services, and this included all but one of those with severe MR. In adult prevalence studies, it is the people who continued to receive services who have been the almost exclusive focus of previous research. Very little attention has been given to the other half, who disappear from MR services after leaving school. As Gruenberg (1964) said (see Chapter 2), either those who disappear from services are doing well and we need to question how we define MR, or they are doing poorly and we are not providing them with the services they need.

Gruenberg's questions about the nature of mild MR have important public policy implications, and they were influential in the design of the present study. In later chapters, we will examine the functioning of those who disappeared from MR services after leaving school and will compare them in various adult roles with peers of the same age and sex from similar social backgrounds.

Figure 5.11 shows a schematic representation of prevalence based on various definitions at different ages up to 22. The theoretical psychometric prevalence of mental retardation is approximately 24 per 1000 based on ≥2 standard deviations below the mean of 100, and represents an IQ below 70. If an IQ of 75 is used as a cut-off, theoretical prevalence would increase. It is well known that the low end of the normal curve of IQ distribution is somewhat enlarged as the

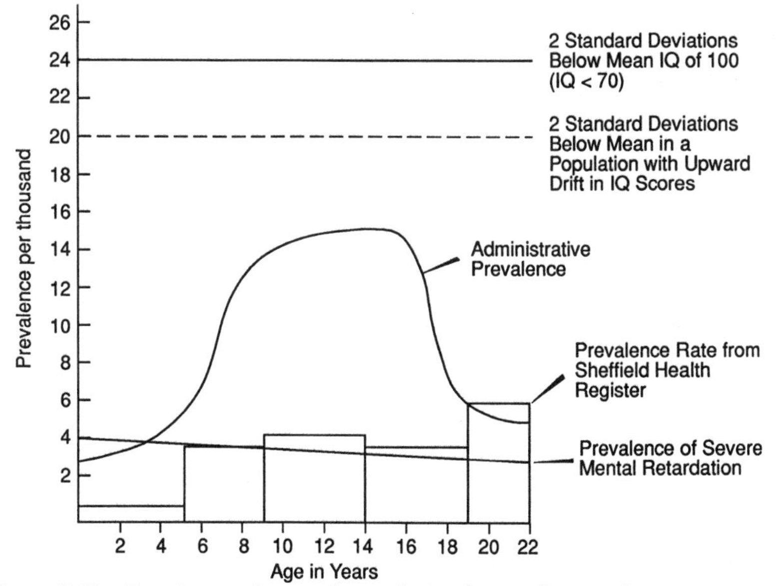

Figure 5.11 Prevalence of mental retardation by age from various sources.

result of impairments of the central nervous system, and this also contributes to an increase in the overall prevalence of mental retardation. The 3 percent prevalence of MR widely cited for many years was based on these considerations. If IQ tests are equivalent across ages, the psychometric prevalence would remain relatively constant, dropping only as the result of mortality.

When the characteristics of the population tested differ from the characteristics of the population on which the test was standardized, departures from the theoretical psychometric prevalence of MR occur. A departure is likely to occur if the social class distribution is different; prevalence increases if the tested population has an unusually high proportion from the lower social classes. Over time, there is evidence of an upward drift in performance of IQ tests, and this will result in a fall in psychometric prevalence.

The adaptive behavior component of MR is based on minimum societal expectations for role performance, and these change during the various stages of life. Expectations for children and for adults differ sharply. During the school years, minimum standards for performance are uniform and become more stringent as the child grows older. In the postschool years, however, these uniform standards are replaced by more variable ones based on the particular role an adult plays.

The age-specific administrative prevalence of those with IQ's below 70–75 is suggested in Figure 5.11. It increases during the school years and drops by approximately one-half after school-leaving age. We examined the prevalence rates of MR obtained from registers kept by the Department of Health in the United Kingdom, which give lower prevalence rates than the administrative classification rates. The data in Figure 5.11 are taken from the Sheffield Health Register (Bayley 1973), where the results were reported for five-year periods and show an increase in the postschool years, unlike age-specific rates based on school placement.

Virtually all the reported variability in prevalence rates occurred in the mild MR range. As Fryers (1987) has pointed out, all those with IQ's below 50 demonstrate severe impairments of adaptive behavior, so IQ is a sufficient criterion for defining severe MR. In Figure 5.11, we provide an approximate median of results obtained, and with age there was a slow decline in rates due to mortality. In recent years, with the adoption of normalization and mainstreaming policies and restrictions on IQ testing, it is extraordinarily difficult to determine the true prevalence rates for mild MR.

6

Clues to Etiology

According to an early etiological classification, mental retardation (MR) comprised two categories: organic and cultural-familial. Organic factors were thought to cause severe MR, and cultural-familial factors mild MR, and we will briefly review conceptual and research developments relating to each of them. Organic factors ("nature") are the result of brain dysfunction from various causes and include injuries, infection, toxins, simple specific gene or chromosome disorders (which can occur in successive generations), and complex genetic factors that determine the endowment for intelligence. Cultural-familial factors ("nurture") are social environmental conditions that influence children's psychosocial development. The relative emphasis given to "nature" and "nurture" as possible causes of mental retardation has varied over time. Eugenics theory, based on proportional inheritance of characteristics such as intelligence, was first postulated by Francis Galton in 1883. Early in the twentieth century, a large research program mounted in the United States produced results purported to support this theory. The eugenics theory was used to justify segregating individuals with mental retardation and state laws requiring the sterilization of women with mental retardation in institutions. The theory led to the advocacy of selective breeding but was later called into question. In 1919 Walter Fernald stated at a meeting, "A dozen years ago, we had practically settled all the problems of 'feeblemindedness.' We had decided that the feeble-minded were all of hereditary origin, that they were pretty much all vicious and depraved and immoral, that they were not capable of self-support. Now there are a number of reasons not to be so sure" (quoted in Kevles 1984c, p. 128).

After World War II, the eugenics theory fell into further disrepute, in part because of the terrible ramifications of the racial policies of Nazi Germany. Nevertheless, familial mental retardation has been recognized for many years. There are some families in which multiple male members have mental retardation, while females are less affected as carriers. Now it is recognized that many, perhaps a majority, of family members with X-linked mental retardation express a "fragile site" on the X chromosome (fragile-X syndrome). The identification of this and other genetic markers has made it possible to examine the frequency of some intergenerational genetic disorders in populations of persons with mental retardation.

In the 1930s, researchers began to examine how social environmental factors contributed to mental retardation. Skeels and his colleagues, for example, published studies on the positive effects of a socially stimulating environment on the children's intelligence (Skeels 1966; Skeels and Dye 1939; Skeels et al. 1938). In the late 1950s, in the Brookland's experiment, Tizard (1964) showed the beneficial effects of moving children with mental retardation from a traditional institution to a residential unit run on more advanced principles of child care. More recently, the Milwaukee Project (Garber 1988) examined the prevention of mental retardation in children at risk through intervention aimed at providing early stimulation for children and training mothers in child care techniques. The results, however, were equivocal. In a review of polygenic and environmental interactions, Clarke (1985) concluded that evidence that psychosocial deprivation alone could cause mental retardation is scant. She continued, "behavioral geneticists agree about the importance of the environment interacting with the genetic template as it becomes activated over time, and that in severely disadvantaged environments development may be considerably retarded . . . [and] . . . children with relatively poor heritability for intelligence may have the additional disadvantage of being raised in suboptimal environments" (pp. 284–286). Separating out the causal roles played by heritable and environmental factors is clearly a complex and difficult task.

The extent to which inheritance of the "low end of the range" of intelligence is a contributor to mental retardation is not known because there are no direct measures. What evidence we have is inferential, based on correlational studies of the IQ's of parents and their offspring and on assumptions following from the Gaussian distribution of IQ proposed by Penrose (1949).

Biomedical Factors

There has long been an interest in biomedical (organic) factors that have etiological implications for mental retardation. A large number of such possible causes have been investigated over the years, and epidemiological inquiries have sought to determine their frequency in populations of individuals with mental retardation. These studies vary in a number of ways.

1. Factors with etiologic implications selected for study have varied depending on the interest of the investigator and the data available. They are also closely related to the time at which the study was done. For example, fetal alcohol syndrome and various other drug-related embryopathies have only recently been implicated as causes of mental retardation. Some studies are restricted to a class of factors, such as obstetrical or genetic, while others have a wider focus.
2. Results will be influenced by the quality of the data, the completeness of ascertainment of children defined as having MR in the population, and the prevalence of MR in the population studied. Especially for mild MR, prevalence rates vary widely, and a high prevalence rate is likely to yield a smaller proportion of biomedical factors than a low prevalence rate.
3. The ages at which children with mild MR are studied will influence prevalence rates (see Chapter 5), which, in turn, will influence the results. Most children with severe MR are identified before they enter school, while children with mild MR are identified more frequently after they enter school, between the ages of 5 and 12. Unless populations are studied up to age 12 or beyond, it is likely that some children with mild MR will be missed. In our follow-up study, all children administratively classified as having MR at any age up to 16 years were identified.

4. The proportion of a given study population for whom some biomedical factor is ascertained varies. Most studies have dealt with severe MR, and the proportion with known biomedical causes has increased over time, as more disorders have been discovered. Fryers (1984) estimated that 80 percent of children currently identified as having severe MR can be given a diagnosis with etiologic implications. In earlier studies, proportions were lower. Studies of biomedical causes of mild MR have been few, but recently they have increased in number. Depending on the definition used, approximately 40 percent of mild MR has a recognized biomedical origin (Hagberg et al. 1981b; Lamont and Dennis 1988).
5. Studies might be expected to vary in the proportions of the population with different biomedical factors, even if all other attributes of the studies could be held constant. For example, the probability of having a child with Down syndrome increases with maternal age, but the proportion of older women bearing children varies from place to place and over time. The use of prenatal diagnosis, such as amniocentesis, and selective abortion, vary by community.

The criteria used to decide which biomedical factors have etiologic implications for mental retardation are based on the frequency with which mental retardation is found among children with a given diagnosis. For example, with few exceptions, children with Down syndrome will have some degree of mental retardation. The presence of cerebral palsy (CP) increases the likelihood that a child will have mental retardation, yet around half of all children with CP do *not* have mental retardation. Somewhat different reasoning may be used in making causal inferences for children known to have mental retardation. When a child has both mental retardation and CP, it may be inferred that the central nervous system impairment that caused the CP also caused the mental retardation. Another example is autism, where approximately 70 percent have IQ's below 70 (Denckla and James 1991). It is now generally accepted that autism has a biologic basis (Folstein and Piven 1991). For children with mental retardation and autism, it may be inferred that the biomedical factor that caused autism also caused the mental retardation.

We are, then, dealing with biomedical factors for which the causal relationships vary, although all have some degree of etiological implication for mental retardation. We reviewed previous studies giving the frequencies of selected biomedical categories with etiological implications for MR among populations of children with severe and mild MR, and these are shown in Table 6.1. Because Fryers (1984) has done a careful review of some of the biomedical categories, we include in the table his estimates of the frequency of CP and epilepsy.

Because of the shortage of epidemiological studies of autism among children with MR, we calculated the frequency of autism for a total population of children with all levels of severity of MR from studies of autism in general populations. Sugiyama, Takei, and Tokuichiro (1992) summarized the general studies. These show prevalence rates of 4–5 per 10,000 in Western studies and 14–15 per 10,000 in Japanese studies. In a recent review, Denckla and James (1991) estimated that 70 percent of autistic individuals had MR, defined as an IQ of less than 70. Based on these figures, the general population would include 3–10 per 10,000 children with autism and mental retardation. To determine how many of the 3 to 10 children with autism and MR would be found in populations of children with MR, the denominator must be reduced to the number of children with MR in the general population. Using the estimate of 12 per 1000 (Richardson and Koller 1985) as the prevalence rate for MR with IQ of less than 70, there would be 12 × 10 = 120 children with MR in a general population of 10,000. In a population of children with MR, there would be 2.5 to 8.3 percent with autism.

Psychosocial Adversity

In general, research into biomedical and cultural-familial factors have proceeded along separate lines of inquiry, but a few studies have examined both (Stein and Susser 1960; Birch et al. 1970; Cooper and Lackus 1984; Lamont and Dennis 1988). Birch et al. (1970) illustrates this approach, using the measure of social class as an indirect indicator of psychosocial adversity. (For an explanation of the social class ratings, see Chapter 14.) For a carefully selected population of children with MR resident in a city at a given time, data were collected on IQ, the family's social class, and whether or not a standardized neurological examination found evidence of central nervous system (CNS) damage. Table 6.2 shows the extent to which children with

Table 6.1 Percentages with selected biomedical diagnoses from other studies of children with IQ <50 and 50–69

	Cerebral palsy		Postnatal injury		Autism		Epilepsy		Down	
Author and date	IQ <50	IQ 50–69	IQ <50	IQ 50–69	IQ <50	IQ 50–69	IQ <50	IQ 50–69	IQ <50	IQ 50–69
Gustavson et al. 1977b	18						30		32	
McDonald 1973	13		8–11				13		23	
Drillien, Jameson, and Wilkinson 1966	12	6.7		3		1.2	8	7.6	32[a]	1.9
Iivanainen 1981	41									
Blomquist et al. 1981		7		4.3 m 0.0 f						6
Hagberg et al. 1981b		9		2				12		2
Corbett 1981							32			
Wald et al. 1977							22			
Bunday, Thake, Todd 1989								3.4		5.7
Czeizel et al. 1980				5.5				5		3
Lamont and Dennis 1988				5				5		1.2
Gillberg et al. 1986					8	4				
Fryers 1984	20–40 (est.)		9–11				20–30 (est.)		26[b]	
Martindale et al. 1988			7.4–12.3						23	
Elwood and Darragh 1981									27	
Einfeld 1984									17.3	
Murphy et al. 1995	28	6					32	7		

a. IQ <55.
b. In annual cohorts from 1967 to 1980, the percentages ranged from 15 to 42 percent with a mean of 26 percent.

Table 6.2 Social class distribution of children with and without evidence of CNS damage who had mild MR and severe MR, presented as actual/expected number

IQ	CNS status	Social class[a]				
		I–IIIa	IIIb	IIIc	IV	V
IQ <50	CNS+	1.03	0.74	1.28	0.97	1.03
IQ 50+	CNS+	0.14	1.01	0.78	0.60	3.80
IQ 50+	CNS−	0.00	0.27	1.22	2.20	3.10
IQ 60+	CNS−	0.00	0.00	1.00	2.40	3.70

Source: Data from Birch et al. 1970, chap. 6, esp. pp. 69, 70, and 71.

Note: A figure greater than 1.0 indicates a higher concentration, and a figure less than 1.0 indicates a lower concentration of cases than expected.

a. See Chapter 7 for explanation of social class.

IQ's above and below 50, with (CNS+) and without (CNS−) CNS damage, were over- or underrepresented in each social class. From the data in Table 6.2, the authors made the following inferences.

IQ < 50, CNS+. "Our finding that these . . . children are randomly distributed across social classes provides no reasonable basis for inferring that social-environmental or familial-constitutional factors had made a significant contribution to the production of handicap" (p. 68).

IQ 50+, CNS+. "The prevalence in Social Class V . . . was 25 times greater than for Social Classes I to IIIa. These findings suggest either that an IQ of 50 or greater deriving from biological insult is less frequent in the highest social class grouping or that given levels of biological insult interact with different social-environmental and family conditions to produce significant subnormality in socially deprived individuals and have little effect on the socially advantaged individuals" (p. 68).

IQ 50+, CNS−. "These data reveal a marked social class gradient, beginning with a total absence of cases in Social Classes I to IIIa, and a stepwise increase in prevalence down the social class scale until a prevalence that is three times greater than expectancy is found in Social Class V. This finding supports the inference that social-environmental and familial factors are contributing to cause in this type of mental subnormality" (p. 70).

Birch et al. (1970) also showed that, for children with IQ's of 60 and above, the skewing toward the lower end of the social class scale was even more extreme (see Table 6.2). After some further analyses of the living conditions of families of children with MR and IQ's of 60 and above and no evidence of CNS damage in Social Classes IV and V, the authors concluded, "While clearly, social environment must exercise a strong influence on the motivations, achievement, and development of the child, we cannot, on the basis of the present study, answer the crucial question as to how these background factors are translated into levels of ability or how they interact with other biologic or genetic influences" (Birch et al. 1970, p. 90).

The Follow-up Study

The main purpose of this chapter is to examine three classes of factors that have etiological implications for mental retardation in the study population:

1. Biomedical factors, including single gene or chromosomal disorders that were recognized in the study children and did not affect multiple generations of the family.
2. Intergenerational genetic disorders, hereafter called family pedigree (since they were derived from the family history rather than directly measured).
3. Psychosocial adversity, the etiological implications of which may not be as clear as for the other two classes of factors.

Of the 221 children who made up the total population of children with mental retardation, some had to be omitted from the present analysis because of missing data. Data on family pedigree were available for 86 percent, on psychosocial adversity on 87 percent, and on biomedical factors for 96 percent. Measures on all three classes of factors were available for 74 percent. The data were derived from interview, observational, and record sources (see Chapter 4). We reviewed these data sources and carried out cross-checks whenever possible. We used many of the diagnoses given in the records; others we derived from descriptions of symptoms.

Biomedical Factors

The biomedical categories and how they were defined are as follows:

Single generation genetic disorders. These included Down syndrome and other recognized single gene or chromosome disorders.

Cerebral malformation. This was an occipital encephelocele.

Identifiable and nonidentifiable dysmorphic syndromes (likely associated with cerebral dysgenesis). The cohort was examined on a number of occasions by pediatricians and pediatric neurologists. Several children had "significantly dysmorphic appearance" to all examiners, without any recognizable syndrome. These children very likely had an underlying biomedical cause for their mental retardation, although it was not specifically identified by syndrome label.

Cerebral palsy. This was defined as chronic motor handicap (that is, more than hyperreflexia) not explainable by peripheral disorder, such as club foot.

Microcephaly. This was defined as head circumference more than two standard deviations below age/sex norms (Nellhaus 1968), or agreement by comments of all professional observers.

Macrocephaly. This was defined as head circumference more than two standard deviations above age/sex norms (Nellhaus 1968), or agreement by comments of all professional observers.

Autism. This diagnosis was not made contemporaneously, but was agreed upon after a review of all data by two clinicians experienced in this area. Because the diagnosis was based on behavioral descriptions by third parties who had not themselves identified the disorder, any uncertainty excluded this diagnosis.

Epilepsy. This was defined as more than one unprovoked seizure.

Birth weight small for gestational age (SGA). A birth weight lower than the tenth percentile for gestational age was classified as SGA (Lubchenko, Hansman, and Boyd 1966).

Attributable postnatal insult and ongoing injury. These included brain injury of an ongoing nature and therefore uncertain timing, including untreated hypothyroidism or brain tumor, and a history of brain injury sufficient to cause mental retardation occurring after twenty-eight days of life and before IQ was measured or outcome assessed. Histories included:

1. Serious head injury with significant loss of function immediately following
2. Meningitis or encephalitis (for example, following measles, tuberculosis, influenza)
3. Encephalopathies of known (for example, uremic) or unknown mechanism (for example, "epileptic encephalopathy," such as

infantile spasms with previous history that child was normal or postictal hemiplegia syndrome)

Not included were histories of brain injury that occurred after twenty-eight days of life and were judged insufficient or inappropriately timed to have caused the mental retardation (although the parent reported that it had), such as skull fractures without major loss of consciousness or injuries occurring after the mental retardation had been recognized. Perinatal asphyxia was omitted, since this remains difficult to diagnose accurately and has been shown to be of low risk for mental retardation in the absence of cerebral palsy. Prematurity was also omitted for similar reasons. Some biomedical disorders, such as fetal alcohol syndrome, were omitted because systematic and contemporaneous data were unavailable. Other evidence of biomedical factors, such as minor dysmorphic features or clumsiness, were not included, because of the subjective nature of the observation and lack of agreement in the literature as to the relevance of such findings.

The concept that various diagnostic factors have different probabilities of causing mental retardation has not been present in the literature, although the extent to which etiologic inferences may be made tend to vary depending on the particular diagnostic factor. An exception to this is Drillien, Jameson, and Wilkinson (1966), who made the distinctions of definite, probable, possible, and uncertain. In our follow-up study, for each of the biomedical factors we assigned a level of probability based on its known associations with mental retardation. A *high* probability was assigned to cerebral palsy, microcephaly, attributable postnatal insult or ongoing injury, Down syndrome, other genetic disorders having a recognized association with mental retardation, autism, and an externally recognizable cerebral malformation (occipital encephalocele). A *medium* probability was assigned to epilepsy, birth weight small for gestational age, macrocephaly, "significantly dysmorphic appearance," and a recognized teratogen exposure where the mother was an insulin-dependent diabetic. There were four children with a medical diagnosis but no clear basis for assigning a probable biomedical cause of the MR: one with an XYY sex chromosome finding (where a causal role for mental retardation is unlikely), another with Wilson's disease (which affects the basal ganglia and impairs communication but should not of itself lead to cognitive impairment), and two with nonattributable head injuries.

Family Pedigree

We did not obtain direct genetic markers of intergenerational disorders in the follow-up study. Instead, we assessed the probability of intergenerational transmission on the basis of the proportion of the child's relatives who had mental retardation (defined as having received MR services).

X-Linked MR, Including Fragile-X Syndrome

X-linked MR was considered *likely* when (1) at least 75 percent of the male siblings (a minimum of two) had MR, and clinical features of the syndrome (macrocephaly, severe MR, autistic or hyperactive behavior) were present in some; or (2) there was a definite X-linkage pattern in the pedigree (son ± brothers ± mother + maternal uncles or cousins) and no other biologic "cause" was present. A *possible* rating was given when (1) at least 50 percent of the male siblings (a minimum of two) had MR; (2) a mother and a single son both had MR; or (3) two male siblings (<50 percent) had both MR *and* clinical characteristics (see above), and there were no other biologic or *likely* genetic "causes" present. Females in the study were included and given a *possible* rating if their male siblings met these criteria.

Other Familial Genetic Disorders

Other familial genetic disorders (mainly of autosomal dominant inheritance) were considered *likely* when almost all (at least four of five) of the members of at least one generation had MR without an X-linked pattern. A *possible* rating was given when MR was present in more than two first- degree relatives over two generations (and no other "cause" was evident).

The terms "likely" and "possible" were necessary because family histories were used as the basis for the diagnosis. Had direct genetic markers been available for the children in the study, a "high" probability of biomedical cause would have been warranted.

Psychosocial Adversity

Psychosocial adversity is more likely to occur among children from the lower end of the social class scale, and the predominance of children with mild MR in lower social class families suggests that psychosocial adversity makes some contribution to mild MR. As we show in Chapter 5, the social class distributions of severe and mild MR in our study are generally in accord with previous research. Severe MR does not show any clear trend across social class; its prevalence is highest, however, in Social Class V. For mild MR, the prevalence rates show a stepwise increase from upper to lower social class.

Social class provides a general measure from which to make some inferences about the lifestyles of families. As Chapter 14 shows, low social class bears some relationship to psychosocial adversity. One alternative to using social class as an indicator of psychosocial adversity is to specify elements in children's social environment that are causally related to mild MR. At the present time the knowledge that would make this possible is insufficient. Jenson (1981) writes,

> My hunch is that the non-genetic variance in IQ is the result of such a myriad of micro-environmental events as to make it extremely difficult, if not impossible, to bring more than a small fraction of these influences under experimental control. The result of all such attempts to date would seem to be consistent with this interpretation.

This leaves the alternative of a more general measure of psychosocial adversity. We used a measure of family stability, which we felt had a closer conceptual relationship to psychosocial adversity than social class. While we consider the family stability measure to be a good indicator of psychosocial adversity, we recognize that psychosocial adversity may not always reflect the micro-environmental influences to which Jensen refers.

The following five-point scale (Richardson, Koller, and Katz 1985a) of family stability ranges from stable to unstable :

1. A *stable* family environment was defined as one in which the childhood years were spent with both parents, who were in at least moderately good health; the father was employed with reasonable steadiness; the mother may or may not have worked outside the home. No aberrant or disturbed behavior was noted in the parents, and there was no evidence that the child was not well cared for.
2. A *less stable* family environment was defined as one in which a child was cared for continuously by at least one parent and

there was no evidence that the child was not well taken care of; however, the family had to cope with the death or desertion of one parent, separation or divorce, or the chronic illness or disability of one or both parents; also present were conditions that were not quite as favorable as those defined in category 1.

3. A *stressful* family environment was defined as one in which it was unclear whether or not the child was well cared for. Death or desertion of both parents may have occurred and, if so, the child may have been raised by other family members or foster parents for the remainder of the time. The child may have been placed in the care of local authority for a short period of time due to the lack of a caretaker. Also included were conditions that were not quite as favorable as defined in category 2, and some family discord or disorganization was present.
4. A *discordant or disorganized* family environment was defined as one in which the child was not well cared for, but there was no intervention by authorities because of abuse or neglect. The child might have been placed in the care of authorities, however, because a caretaker was lacking or had left; the child was then brought up in a foster family with intermediate care by local authorities.
5. A *markedly unstable* environment is one in which the child was abused, neglected, or abandoned. Family disorganization, disruptions, and discord were present. Parents were incompetent or had disturbed behavior, necessitating intervention by authorities. The child's upbringing was marked by instability and uncertainty and often included a series of different caretakers.

All the evidence available from multiple data sources was used in rating each child on family stability. It should be noted that MR in other family members was not taken into account in this rating and that it was carried out independently of the measure of family pedigree.

The measure of family stability provides a reasonable basis for inferring the degree of psychosocial adversity, but it should be considered a probability measure. When using this measure, we found that children with a family stability rating of 3 to 5 had a far higher frequency of adult behavior disturbance than children with a family stability rating of 1 or 2 (Richardson, Koller, and Katz 1985c). This dichotomy provides a reasonable basis for considering a rating of 3 to 5 as an indicator of psychosocial adversity.

Biomedical Factors—Follow-up Study

In the follow-up study, biomedical factors were present for 80 percent of children with severe MR and 34 percent of those with mild MR. From previous studies, it has been estimated that 80 percent of children with severe MR, and 40 percent with mild MR have biomedical etiological factors present (Fryers 1984; Hagberg et al. 1981b; Lamont and Dennis 1988). Our results are thus in accord with more recent research. Table 6.3 shows the frequency of various diagnoses at different IQ levels. First, we will examine *high-probability* factors.

Cerebral palsy, the most frequent high-probability diagnosis, was found in 40/213 (18 percent) of all the young people with MR. The frequency within each IQ group was highest for those with IQ's below 50 and generally decreased in frequency as IQ increased. Cerebral palsy, together with other high-probability diagnoses, also occurred most frequently in individuals with IQ's below 50, and these multiple diagnoses also decreased as IQ increased.

Microcephaly, the second most frequently occurring high-probability diagnosis, was found in 20/213 (9 percent) of the study population and occurred five times more frequently in individuals with severe MR. There was a striking contrast in the frequency by IQ with which microcephaly occurred as a single factor and in combination with other high-probability factors. Among children with mild MR (IQ 50 and above), microcephaly always occurred alone and may well be a primary developmental condition not associated with brain injury, whereas among those with severe MR (IQ <50), 83 percent of children with microcephaly had multiple high-probability factors. Microcephaly in children with severe MR is often the result of severe brain injury or maldevelopment, and is therefore "incidental" to another etiology of MR.

Down syndrome occurred in 11/213 (5 percent) of the study population and 10/11 had IQ's below 50. It was more frequent as a single high-probability diagnosis than any other.

Postnatal injury was found in 13/213 (6 percent) of the study population, and its frequency was not related to IQ level. It was often present in combination with other high-probability biomedical factors.

Table 6.3 Biomedical diagnoses by level of probability and IQ group

	IQ <50 (*n* = 46)	IQ 50–59 (*n* = 46)	IQ 60–69 (*n* = 74)	IQ 70+ (*n* = 47)	Total (*n* = 213)[a]
A. *High Probability—Biomedical*					
Cerebral palsy	17 (59)[b]	6 (33)	13 (23)	4 (0)	40
Microcephaly	12 (83)	3 (0)	2 (0)	3 (0)	20
Down syndrome	10 (30)	1 (0)	0	0	11
Genetic (other than Down)	1 (100)	1 (100)	2 (50)	0	4
Postnatal insult	7 (57)	3 (67)	2 (100)	1 (0)	13
Autism	6 (83)	2 (50)	1 (100)	1 (0)	10
Cerebral malformation	1 (0)	0	0	0	1
B. *Medium Probability—Biomedical*					
Epilepsy	16 (100)	8 (75)	7[c] (29)	2 (0)	33
Small/gestational age	0	1 (0)	6[c] (0)	4 (50)	11
Macrocephaly	2 (50)	0	0	1 (0)	3
Dysmorphic syndrome	0	3 (0)	1 (0)	1 (0)	5
Teratogen (IDDM)	0	1 (0)	0	0	1
C. *Pedigree*					
X-linked MR likely	1 (0)	0	4 (0)	2 (0)	7
Other pedigree likely	1 (100)	4 (0)	2 (0)	1 (100)	8
X-linked MR possible	2 (100)	4 (25)	8 (25)	7 (14)	21
Other pedigree possible	0	1 (0)	3 (0)	2 (50)	6

a. There were inadequate data for this analysis for eight cases.
b. Figures in parentheses show the percentage with additional high probability diagnosis.
c. One child had both SGA and epilepsy.

Autism was found in 10/213 (5 percent) of the population. It was most frequent among those with severe MR, where, with one exception, other high-probability factors were also present.

Cerebral malformation was found in only one child with severe MR, and no other high-probability factors were present.

The following factors were given *medium probability.*

Epilepsy, by far the most frequent medium probability diagnosis, was present in 33/215 (15 percent) of the population. All children with epilepsy who had IQ's below 50 also had a high-probability diagnosis, but this occurred with decreasing frequency as IQ increased.

Small for gestational age, the second most frequent medium probability factor at 11/213 (5 percent), was found only in children with mild MR.

The remaining categories, dysmorphic syndrome and a single teratogen, occurred only in the mild MR range; none of these children also had an additional high-probability biomedical diagnosis.

In Table 6.4 we compare our results dealing with biomedical factors (shown in Table 6.3) with a summary of results from other studies. Our rates for cerebral palsy are at the upper end of the range. While this may be a true comparison, it may also, in part, be so because cases were missed in other studies, or because we included cases of mild cerebral palsy omitted from some of the other studies.

Postnatal injury rates in our study are slightly higher than those in other studies.

Down syndrome rates are in the mid-range of results from other studies for severe MR, but they are at the low end of the range for mild MR. Children with Down syndrome in our study population were sometimes institutionalized at an early age; those kept at home were excluded from the special school for children with MR and placed instead in a Junior Occupation Center (see Chapter 15). Had these children been given more favorable circumstances for their social and intellectual development, some of them might have been in the mild MR range.

The percentage of epilepsy in our follow-up study is at the high end of the range for both mild and severe MR compared to other studies. One explanation may be that the study followed children to age 22, thus spanning more years than other studies. We know that for some young people in our follow-up study (see Chapter 9) the onset of epilepsy did not occur until the late teen years.

Autism was most frequent in the young people with severe MR (13 percent), and its occurrence decreased in frequency as IQ increased. Although we were unable to find an epidemiological study of autism,

Table 6.4 Percentages with which diagnostic categories were found in the follow-up and other studies

	IQ <50		IQ 50–69	
Diagnostic categories	Follow-up study	Est. from other studies	Follow-up study	Est. from other studies
Cerebral palsy	37	12–41	16	7–9
Postnatal injury	15	7–12	4	2–5
Down syndrome	22	17–33	1	1–6
Epilepsy	35	8–36	13	3–12

we were able to make an estimate (see above) from other research of between 2.5 and 8.3 percent for all levels of severity of MR. Our study result of 5 percent fits within this range.

Family Pedigree

For comparative purposes, we consider that fragile-X syndrome comprised most X-linked disorders. Previous studies of fragile-X syndrome are summarized in Table 6.5. The rates for severe MR range between 4 percent and 5 percent; for mild MR, the range is far greater and, when genders are combined, extends from less than 1 percent to 8 percent. For severe MR, our rate is 3 percent for likely probability, compared to the 4 percent to 5 percent of other studies. For mild MR, we used an upper IQ limit of 69 to be comparable with other studies and found rates of 3 percent for probable and 4 percent for possible. This is within the 3 percent to 7 percent range in rates found in other studies.

Table 6.5 Percentages with fragile-X syndrome from other studies of children with IQ <50 and 50–69

	Percentage with fragile-X syndrome[a]	
Author and date	IQ <50	IQ 50–69
Bunday et al. 1985	4	3.6 m
		6.0 f
Thake et al. 1987	4.8 m	6.4 m
	4.3 f	9.6 f
Gustavson, Holmgren, and Blomquist, 1987		3
Turner, Daniel, and Frost 1980		1.5 m
		6.9 f
Blomquist et al. 1983		8.3 m
		0.0 f
Lamont, Dennis, and Seabright 1986		0.0 m
		1.4 f
Brown et al. Estimated from 1987		10

a. Likely fragile-X-linked MR in the present study and clinically determined fragile-X syndrome in other studies. For all mental retardation, 3–10 percent is the estimated range (see text).

Psychosocial Adversity

We have used family instability as an indicator of psychosocial adversity and may regard it as a probable measure. Family instability was experienced by children with IQ's of 60 and above more than twice as frequently as by children with IQ's below 60 (IQ 70+, 49 percent; IQ 60–69, 51 percent; IQ 50–59, 22 percent; IQ <50, 21 percent). Because there are no other epidemiological studies of psychosocial adversity, no comparisons can be made.

Etiological Factors Alone and in Combination

Our follow-up study provided a unique opportunity to determine the frequency with which the three sets of etiological factors were present singly, or in various combinations, for children with MR. To do so we needed data on all three factors for each child, and these data were available for 28/46 (61 percent) of those with severe MR and 136/175 (78 percent) of those with mild MR.

We combined the various biomedical diagnoses into two categories—high and medium probability—to make the analysis manageable. Among all the children with MR, 47 percent had some high probability diagnosis and 11 percent had only a medium probability diagnosis. Among those with severe MR, high probability biomedical factors were found most often, whereas among children with mild MR, medium probability factors were present more often.

Among the children with severe MR, we were unable to find evidence of any of the three factors among 4 of the 28 children with severe MR for whom we had complete data. For the remaining 24, all but one had a high probability biomedical diagnosis; the one exception had a diagnosis of moderate probability. For 18/24 (75 percent), the biomedical factor occurred alone. Among the six remaining, half also had evidence of psychosocial adversity; for the other half, all three factors were present. The findings are in agreement with previous research showing that biomedical factors play a dominant role in severe MR. None of those with severe MR had psychosocial adversity as a single factor. This agrees with Clarke's (1985) conclusion that severe MR resulting from psychosocial adversity is extremely rare. For the four cases in which none of the three factors was present, it is likely that some possibly yet unknown biomedical factor was present.

Table 6.6 shows the etiological factors found among those with mild MR. For ease of analysis, we combined biomedical categories of high and medium probability, and family pedigree of likely and possible probability. We then examined whether the etiological factors differed for the IQ categories of 50–59, 60–69, and 70+. Numbers were small, but significant differences were found, although there was somewhat more psychosocial adversity above IQ 60 and more biomedical factors below 60. These IQ groups were therefore combined. We were unable to find any of the three etiological factors for 23 percent of the children. Each of the three factors contributed, alone or in combination, to the following extent: psychosocial adversity (63/136, 46 percent), followed by biomedical factors (46/136, 34 percent) and family pedigree (35/136, 26 percent).

Table 6.6 Frequency of the three classes of etiological factors as they occurred singly and in combination among the population with mild mental retardation

	Population with Mild MR		
	Number		Percentage
No Etiological Factor Found		31	23
Single Factors			
Biomedical			
High probability	17	30	22
Moderate probability	13		
Family pedigree			
Likely	1	9	7
Possible	8		
Psychosocial adversity		28	21
Two Factors			
Biomedical (High) + Family Pedigree (Likely)	1	3	2
Biomedical (High) + Family Pedigree (Possible)	2		
Biomedical (High) + Psychosocial Adversity	6	12	9
Biomedical (Moderate) + Psychosocial Adversity	6		
Family Pedigree (Likely) + Psychosocial Adversity	11	22	16
Family Pedigree (Possible) + Psychosocial Adversity	11		
Three Factors			
Biomedical (High) + Family Pedigree (Possible) + Psychosocial Adversity	1		<1
TOTAL	136		100
Excluded because of missing data	39		

Psychosocial adversity appears to play a lesser etiological role in mild MR than was previously thought. As a single factor, it was present in only 21 percent, less than the 34 percent found in combination with other factors. Not all children who experience psychosocial adversity have mental retardation. For those who do, this may be due to a combination of psychosocial adversity and a heritable endowment at the low end of the range of intelligence. At present, there is no way of testing this hypothesis. We found that family pedigree factors rarely occurred alone (7 percent) or in combination with biomedical factors (3 percent).

The frequency with which family pedigree was found in conjunction with psychosocial adversity is striking. When family pedigree had a likely probability, it occurred in combination with psychosocial adversity for 11/13 (85 percent) of the children. When family pedigree had a possible probability, the combination was less frequent (12/22, 55 percent). Because of their likely intellectual impairment, the parents of young people with family pedigrees may have difficulties coping, and may create conditions of psychosocial adversity for their children. When this occurs, the young people with family pedigrees have the double disadvantage of experiencing psychosocial adversity and having the genetic disorder. Biomedical factors are the only ones that occur more frequently alone (22 percent) than with psychosocial (10 percent) and pedigree factors (3 percent).

Earlier, we compared our results on the three factors separately with other studies. Since no previous studies have examined how the three factors combine, we have no basis for comparing these results. The comparisons we were able to make, however, between past epidemiological studies and our follow-up study increase our confidence that our results are not idiosyncratic. The dominant role of biomedical factors with etiological implications for severe MR has been known for some time, and the present study provides additional confirmation. This chapter makes an original contribution to our understanding of the etiology of mild MR. We have attempted to subdivide the concept of "cultural-familial" into the "nurture" component of psychosocial adversity and the "nature" component of intergenerational genetic disorders, which we have called family pedigree.

As in other studies, we were unable to find any causal factors for some portion of the population with MR. This occurred for 14 percent of those with severe MR and 23 percent for those with mild MR. Among some of these, we would postulate that unknown biomedical and family pedigree factors were present, rather than only psychosocial adversity, and to the extent that future research supports this speculation, this would lead to a decrease in the percentage of people with mild MR for whom psychosocial adversity is the only etiological factor known.

Part III

Individual Characteristics

7

Stability and Change in IQ

As far back as 1922 it was noted that, with repeated testing over time, many children showed marked changes in IQ (Baldwin and Stecher 1922). Later, in the California Guidance study, Honzik, McFarlane, and Allen (1948) found that between ages 6 and 18, more than half of the children showed a shift of 15 or more IQ points, about a third a shift of 20 or more IQ points, and a few changes of 30 points or more. No such studies have been carried out, however, on populations with mental retardation.

A problem in all longitudinal studies of IQ is how to differentiate true changes in intellectual functioning from changes that are a function of either expected variation or uncontrolled factors in the test or test administration. The chance of identifying an aberrant score increases if several scores are obtained and a single score is discrepant with the overall series. Greater assurance of true change is possible where there is a steady upward or downward progression in test scores over time, compared to a series of scores that fluctuate up and down over time with no clear slope.

Many investigators have struggled with the problem of how to measure stability and change in IQ. Some of the methods that have been tried are reviewed by Moriarty (1966), Anastasi (1968), Bayley (1970), and Wohlwill (1980). All investigators face the dilemma described by Moriarty (1966): "We hoped to steer a narrow path between the pitfall of dynamically sterile, but methodologically sound, research, and clinically meaningful, but scientifically unverifiable, observation" (p. 40).

Haan (1963) and Moriarty (1966) both suggested that histories of IQ scores be divided into the four categories: scores that increase, decrease, fluctuate, and remain stable. For a population of children with mental retardation, there is no generally accepted convention concerning the size of increases and decreases that denote real change.

The Follow-up Study

The children who were classified as mentally retarded (MR) were tested by an educational psychologist at different ages during the school years using the Terman Merrill (L) and the Stanford-Binet (L-M second revision) tests of intelligence. Scores were generally available for the time of placement in the special school and, periodically thereafter, while the child was at the special school. To examine IQ scores during the school-age years from 5 to 15, the time was divided into three periods: 5 to less than 9, 9 to less than 12, and 12 to 15. For inclusion in the analysis, we required the child's record to have IQ scores in at least two of these age periods. We established this criterion because some children were not classified as MR until the second period and some had no scores in the third period because they had returned to regular school.

The scores in the IQ history of each child were determined and divided into the following categories:

Stable: IQ scores with a range of 0 to 4 points.

Increases and decreases: IQ scores with a steady increase or decrease of 5 or more points.

Fluctuation: IQ scores with no steady increase or decrease and a range of scores of 5 or more points.

Our analysis included 157 children. Excluded were 10 young people who had died and 29 for whom the IQ data were missing. We also excluded 25 children whose IQ's were always below 50 because of the difficulty of obtaining accurate IQ scores below 50.

For 127 children, we obtained IQ scores in all three age periods, and for 28 children, scores for two age periods. We made an exception to the rule requiring scores in two age periods for 2 children with three IQ scores in only one age period. One had an increase of 12 points, the other a decrease of 23 points, and other information indicated that these changes were valid. The median number of tests given was five, the number ranging from two to seven (20 children with two scores, 7 children with seven scores).

History of IQ's

A stable history of IQ scores, with a range of 0 to 4 points across the three time periods, was found for only 10 percent of the children (see Table 7.1). Of the children who showed a directional change, decreases were far more frequent than increases (41 percent and 14 percent, respectively). The remaining 34 percent of the children had fluctuating scores.

Defining a stable history as a range of between 0 and 4 IQ points may be too conservative. The consequences of changing this definition by increments of one additional IQ point is shown in Table 7.1. By increasing the upper limit from four to nine IQ points, the proportion of stable histories increased from 10 percent to 43 percent. Whatever definition of stable is used, there were three to five times as many children whose IQ histories reflected decreases rather than increases.

Among the 62 children whose IQ scores decreased by 5 or more points, 18 ended up with IQ scores below 50. All 18 had decreases in scores of 9 or more points, and the median decrease was 16 points. Only two children had early scores below 50 and later scores above 50, and these were small changes.

Table 7.1 Stability and change in IQ histories during the age period of 5–15 years using different definitions of stability, in percent ($N = 157$)

Definition of stable	Increases	Decreases	Fluctuations	Stable
0–4 points	14	41	34	10
0–5	11	39	33	16
0–6	9	39	32	20
0–7	7	34	30	29
0–8	6	29	26	38
0–9	6	27	24	43

Ages When IQ Changes Occurred

Because IQ scores were available for the majority of the children for the three periods within the overall age range of 5 to 15, we can examine whether the amount of change in scores varied more during earlier or later ages. To do this we divided the age range when the children attended school into three periods: from age 5 to less than 9, from 9 to less than 12, and from 12 to 15. Early changes were defined as those between the first and the second periods, late changes as those between the second and third periods. These changes were of three kinds: increase (IQ change of plus 5 or more); decrease (IQ change of minus 5 or more); and stable (IQ changes from plus or minus 0 to 4 points). The analysis was restricted to the 127 children for whom scores were available for each of the three time periods and omitted the 18 children who were transferred back to regular schools before the third time period, and so had IQ scores for only the earlier period.

A stable score was again defined as a change of not more than four IQ points between two time periods. Table 7.2 shows that the changes in IQ scores occurred predominantly between the first and second periods. Only 27 percent of the scores remained stable, 17 percent

Table 7.2 Stability and change in IQ scores between the first and second periods and between the second and third periods, in percent

Stability and change in IQ scores	Comparison between first two periods: age 5 to less-than-9, and 9 to less-than-12	Comparison between second and third periods: Age to less-than-12, and 12 to 15
Increases		
20+	2	0
10 to 19	4	0
5 to 9	11	6
Stable		
+4 to −4	27	91
Decreases		
5 to 9	27	4
10 to 19	26	
20+	4	
Total *n*	127	127

increased, and 57 percent decreased. By contrast, between the second and third periods, 91 percent had stable scores, and the few children who showed a change were divided almost equally between small increases and small decreases.

The lack of stability in IQ scores during the age period when most of the children were classified as MR poses a dilemma for those responsible for defining children as MR and emphasizes the need for educational authorities to monitor carefully the progress of all children they consider as MR. The histories of the children classified as MR show evidence, for example, in the transfers of children from one kind of educational service to another, that the authorities in Aberdeen did monitor the children's progress. For those children who were transferred from the special school back to regular schools, 41 percent showed increases in scores, and 53 percent had stable scores. Only one child showed a decrease in IQ. By contrast, of the children who were transferred from the special school to the Junior Occupation Center (a program for children unable to cope in the special school), 88 percent showed a decrease in scores, and for half of these, the decrease was 15 or more IQ points. None showed increases in scores. Those who remained at the special school throughout their schooling had a distribution of increases, decreases, and stable IQ scores intermediate between those children who returned to regular schools and those who transferred to the Junior Occupation Center.

The large number of children with IQ changes during the early period of schooling is reason for precluding the use of young children in studies of IQ distributions. There are also questions relating to the reasons for the large declines in IQ. Since they occurred after placement in the special school, it is possible that the placement contributed to the decline. Alternatively, declines at these ages may be a phenomenon of the natural course of MR as demands on the child increase, because the child does not progress at a normal pace. This explanation seems likely, but since no other epidemiological studies have examined the question, it must remain unanswered for now.

At the beginning of this chapter we cited earlier studies that showed marked changes in IQ scores during childhood. In our follow-up study, we also found marked changes over the childhood period, but predominantly in the early school years, and decreases outnumbered increases.

8

Behavior Disturbance

This chapter will examine the following questions:

1. What are the rates of behavior disturbance[1] among young people with mental retardation (MR), and do these rates vary by gender, IQ, age, and type of disturbance?
2. Is behavior disturbance more common among young people with MR than among those without MR? If it is more common, what is the size of the difference and does it vary by gender, IQ, age, and type of disturbance?
3. How much does behavior disturbance change, or remain the same, between childhood and adulthood? Among children with MR, do those with behavior disturbance have a greater risk of behavior disturbance as young adults than those who do not? Does this vary by gender and IQ? What factors contribute to behavior disturbance?

Previous Research

Individuals with and without Mental Retardation

It has long been accepted that behavior disturbance occurs more

1. Many terms for behavior disturbance occur in the literature. These include "emotional disorders," "psychiatric disorders or illness," "mental illness," "deviant behavior," "aberrant or maladaptive behavior," "behavior abnormalities," and "insanity." We will include "behavior disturbance" as a general term to include all these alternatives.

frequently among people with MR than among people without MR. In an early text on MR, Tredgold (1908) estimated that "proneness to insanity" was twenty-six times higher in those with MR than in the ordinary population. The DSM-IV classification (APA 1994) estimated that the prevalence of mental disorders (other than MR) is at least three or four times greater among people with MR than among the general population (p. 42).

There are few studies comparing the frequency of behavior disturbance among people with MR and among the general population. In their Isle of Wight study, Rutter, Tizard, and Whitmore (1970) found rates of behavior disturbance to be 6.8 percent for all children on the island, and 22.4 percent for children with intellectual retardation, some of whom would not have been classified as MR.

Special attention has been paid, however, to antisocial behavior. It was long held, based primarily on eugenic theory, that people with MR had a predisposition for criminal behavior, and these beliefs provided a rationale for institutionalization. Follow-up studies of children with mild MR into their young adult years showed higher rates of antisocial behavior for them than for nonretarded peers (Ramer 1946; Kennedy 1948; Ferguson and Kerr 1960; Baller, Charles, and Miller 1967). These studies were reviewed in Chapter 3, and some of their results must remain questionable because of limitations in the study designs.

There have also been studies of antisocial behavior in general populations that looked at level of intelligence. May (1981) examined the court records of 5,654 boys aged 13 to 17 in Aberdeen, Scotland, and found that the delinquency rate for those with IQ's <90 was 29 percent, compared with 11 percent for boys with IQ's ≥90. In a prospective study on delinquency in London, Farrington and West (1981) found the average nonverbal IQ's of delinquent groups to be 95, and of nondelinquent groups 101, a difference large enough for statistical testing to find low IQ a significant precursor of delinquency. In both these studies, low IQ was one of a constellation of factors associated with delinquent behavior.

Studies that have examined the intelligence levels of prison or offender populations have added to the evidence that individuals with low IQ's have higher rates of antisocial behavior than the population in general. In a review, Santamour and West (1979) reported that studies assessing the intelligence of offender populations gave rates ranging from 9 percent to 27 percent for offenders with IQ's <70. Even though the authors considered the lower rates more accurate, 9 percent was still much higher than the rates of MR in the general population. MacEachron (1979) found reports of an even wider range in prevalence rates of MR in offender populations, and she also considered the higher rates inaccurate. She suggested that the wide variability was due to the use of different population bases and different ways of measuring intelligence. Given her own data on male offenders, MacEachron concluded that the "prevalence rate of mentally retarded adult male offenders is only slightly higher than the prevalence rates of retarded male adults in the general population."

Populations with Mental Retardation

We will confine our attention to behavior disturbance in epidemiological studies, because other types of research have not dealt with representative populations of persons with mental retardation. The bias in institutional studies was described by Gunzburg (1974), who noted that "it is the problem case who will be institutionalized, whilst the adjusted and amenable will be accommodated in the community as long as possible" (p. 709).

Severe Mental Retardation

In community studies of children and adolescents with severe mental retardation, the percentages with behavior disturbance range widely, from 21 percent to 64 percent: 21 percent (Bernassi et al. 1990), 37 percent (Einfield et al. 1992), 41 percent (McQueen et al. 1987), 47 percent (Corbett 1977b), 52 percent (Birch et al. 1970), 64 percent (Gillberg et al. 1986). One study excluded several children whose MR was so severe, a rating of psychiatric status was not possible (Gillberg et al. 1986). In another, 20 percent of the population were given a diagnosis of uncertain (Birch et al. 1970).

A number of explanations may account for these results. Reid (1985) writes, "One of the main dilemmas in establishing prevalence rates for psychiatric disorders in mentally retarded persons arises from the difficulty in defining what constitutes a case. Whereas it is possible to agree on the presence of disorder in more florid examples of psychiatric illness, such as acute mania for example, it becomes far harder to reach a consensus on the milder forms of neurotic personality and behavior problems" (p. 293).

The methods developed for diagnosing general populations have been found to be inappropriate for persons with severe MR. As Reid (1985) further states,

> Psychiatric diagnosis and symptomatology are very substantially language-based, but language development and vocabulary are usually limited in mentally retarded people, and more severely retarded patients frequently have no language at all. There are difficulties, therefore, in gaining access to their thought processes, and to their ways of perceiving and interpreting events . . . At the level of psychiatric symptomatology, phenomena such as thought disorders, hallucinations, delusions, ideas of influence and of significance, all of which are key concepts in the identification of psychiatric illness, are entirely language-bound, and rely on a reasonable level of verbal fluency. (pp. 292–293)

Corbett (1979), who studied behavior disturbance in a population of individuals with severe MR, concluded that "the largest group of people with marked behavior symptoms could not be classified under any of the conventional categories of psychiatric illness or childhood psychoses" (p. 21).

In the studies of severe MR cited above, there was no uniformity in the definitions used; in some, no definitions were given. The studies also differ in whether each person in the population was examined for behavior disturbance or whether record sources were used.

Mild Mental Retardation

In community studies of children and adolescents with mild mental retardation, the percentages with behavior disturbance also vary widely, from 20 percent to 57 percent: 20 percent (Lamont and Dennis 1988), 22.5 percent (Rutter, Graham, and Yule 1970a), 31 percent (Hagberg et al. 1981b), 30 percent (Birch et al. 1970), 57 percent (Gillberg et al. 1986). Gillberg et al., who studied in adolescence the same young people with mild MR who had been studied five years previously by Hagberg et al. (1981b), found nearly twice the rate of behavior disturbance as the earlier study. This may have been the result of changes with age, but it is more likely that their findings differed because Gillberg et al. carried out individual psychiatric examinations, while Hagberg et al. relied on record sources.

In studies of children with mild MR, investigators less often face the difficulty of very limited communication found among children with severe MR. At the same time, full ascertainment of children with mild MR has become increasingly difficult, the borderline area between those with and without mild MR is broad, and investigators differ in their definitions of mild MR. Different definitions of mild MR can result in different rates of behavior disturbance.

Severity of Mental Retardation and Frequency of Behavior Disturbance

Because few of the studies we reviewed examined the whole range of severity of MR, there is no clear indication of differences in the percentages of children with mild MR and those with severe MR who also have behavior disturbance. The two exceptions were Birch et al. (1970) and Gillberg et al. (1986). Both of these studies showed a higher frequency of behavior disturbance among children with severe MR, but both studies also encountered difficulties in making diagnoses.

Studies of general populations of children who do not have MR do show increased risk of behavior disturbance as IQ decreases (Mittelman et al. 1978; Rutter, Tizard, and Whitmore 1970). It does not follow however, that the same association would be found within the IQ range of MR.

Gender Differences

Few of the authors of all the studies we reviewed gave separate results for boys and for girls. Birch et al. (1970) did, but found no significant difference in behavior disturbance between boys and girls with MR. Gillberg et al. (1986) found a slight excess of behavior disturbance in boys among children with mild MR.

Behavior Disturbance in Childhood as a Risk Factor

The prognosis of childhood behavior disturbance through adolescence and into young adulthood is an important concern of parents and human service professionals. In dealing with children with MR, there is heightened reason for concern, for they may be at greater risk of behavior disturbance than others.

There are few studies of behavior disturbance in populations of children followed through into adolescence or adulthood and no follow-up studies of young people with mental retardation. After reviewing the literature, Mellsop (1974) concluded,

> The natural history of psychiatric illness is a subject in which most express interest, many believe they understand, but on which relatively few systematic studies have been published. Despite the widespread conviction that adult behavior patterns are largely laid down in childhood, few attempts have been made to reassess persons seen in childhood when they become adults. Longitudinal studies on children have generally been concerned only with short-term follow-up not extending into adulthood, with small numbers of patients, without adequate controls, or with a highly selected childhood diagnostic group. (p. 689)

Follow-up studies of children who did not have mental retardation indicate that children with behavior disturbance were at higher risk of continued behavior disturbance at older ages than children who did not have behavior disturbance. Mellsop (1974) found that children who experienced psychiatric disorders were at increased risk for adult disorders: "20 years after their referral to the Department of Psychiatry, Royal Children's Hospital, the adults have a four-fold increase over the comparable general population in their risk of being patients of the Victoria (Australia) Mental Health Department" (p. 697).

In a review of relationships between child and adult psychiatric disorders, Rutter (1973) concluded, "Psychopathy is the one disorder which has its roots most firmly set in childhood, with repetitive and widespread antisocial behavior in adult life often leading to later persisting disorders of personality" (p. 685).

In another review, Rutter et al. (1977) described a study of children aged 10 to 11 in the Isle of Wight, who were followed until they were 14 to 15. These children did not have MR. They reported that children with conduct disorders fared worst: three quarters of them were still showing the disorder at follow-up. The outlook for children with emotional disorders was significantly better. Children with both emotional and conduct disorders had an intermediate outcome.

Factors Related to Behavior Disturbance

Brain Dysfunction

It has been proposed that brain dysfunction contributes to both mental retardation and behavior disturbance. Corbett (1977a), although holding a generally biosocial position, concluded from a review that "there is good evidence that children with organic brain dysfunction have a greatly increased susceptibility to psychiatric disorder . . . Virtually all children with an IQ below 50 have demonstrable organic brain disease and this is also true for a substantial minority (20–30%) of mildly retarded children" (p. 853). Shaffer (1977), in contrast, has questioned whether impaired neurological functioning contributes to the higher frequency of behavior disturbance: "It is important to bear in mind the biasing effect of conditions which are known to be associated with psychiatric disorder and which occur more frequently in brain-damaged children . . . Some forms of brain damage . . . occur more often in children from socially and otherwise disadvantaged families. Studies which do not take these factors into account may misleadingly attribute effects to brain injury rather than to sequelae or associations which do not affect all brain damaged children" (p. 185).

Psychosocial Adversity

A number of studies provide evidence of the relationship between psychosocial adversity and behavior disturbance. Nihira, Meyers, and Mink (1980) found that the social adjustment of children with MR was related to cohesiveness and harmony at home. Stein and Susser (1960) examined the childhood experience of individuals with mild MR who were followed up as adults. They found that legal charges, which may be related to antisocial behavior, were more often brought against the adults whose childhood experiences included discontinuities in upbringing and/or care that failed to meet the basic standards expected for children.

In a report on behavior disturbance in adults with MR, Frost (1984) examined a range of factors that might contribute to the development of the disturbance. The major factors identified in the report were parental discord and disorganization, which occurred significantly more often in the families of individuals with behavior disturbance. Werner and Smith (1980), reporting on their longitudinal study of a general population of children in Kauai, Hawaii, found a pronounced lack of emotional support in the homes of most children with serious behavior problems, one that persisted through adolescence.

Reviewing the literature on nonretarded children, Rutter and Madge (1981) found that behavior disturbance occurred more frequently among those whose parents had mental disorders and criminal behavior, and where there was parental discord and disturbance. Furthermore, children who experienced broken homes, parental death, and multiple separations from their primary caretakers were at greater risk of behavior disturbance than were children who did not experience these conditions. They concluded that "a person's personality develops on the basis provided by stable, harmonious relationships in childhood, so that if all a child experiences is discord and distorted relationships he will suffer accordingly" (p. 206).

Using the same methods and definitions, Rutter et al. (1977) carried out community studies of behavior disturbance on the Isle of Wight and in an inner London borough. They found that the children in London had higher rates of behavior disturbance than the children on the Isle of Wight. In examining the reasons for this difference, they concluded that it was largely due to the higher proportion of disadvantaged children in London.

Mental Retardation, Family Stress, and Behavior Disturbance

A child with MR creates stresses in the family that, in turn, contribute to behavior disturbance in the child. Crnic, Friedrick, and Greenberg (1983) reviewed the evidence for this transactional process and pointed out that research on the families of children with MR has had an inherent expectation of "a deleterious or pathological outcome in these families." They conclude, however, that "the ubiquity of such impaired adjustment has certainly come into question" (p. 132). A major shortcoming of the research they reviewed was the lack of information about the children with MR. Often the researchers neither noted the severity of the MR nor provided information on any other kinds of disablement the children might have had. Mercer (1966) proposed that interpersonal stress was related to the burden of care, which depends on the degree of the child's intellectual deficit and the severity and multiplicity of other forms of disability. According to Farber (1968), the higher the socioeconomic status of the family, the greater the impact of labeling a child as mentally retarded on family relationships.

Factors Intrinsic to Mental Retardation

Tarjan (1977) suggested that "retarded individuals are highly vulnerable to emotional traumata. Stresses that result in no significant sequelae in an average child or adult can produce overt psychiatric manifestations in retarded persons" (p. 407). Corbett (1977a) suggested, however, that "although emotional disturbance may occasionally impair intellectual performance, that is not the explanation of the association. Low IQ generally antedates the psychiatric disorder so that the retardation or factors associated with it must lead to psychiatric disorder rather than the other way around" (p. 832).

Nihira, Meyers, and Mink (1980) proposed an interaction between factors intrinsic to mental retardation and extrinsic factors related to the home environment: "since personality development of mentally retarded children is at greater risk because of their retardation, the impact of home environment appears particularly pronounced for this population" (p. 5).

The Follow-up Study

Our follow-up study used four categories of behavior disturbance based on a multiaxial classification of childhood psychiatric disorders developed by Rutter, Shaffer, and Shepherd (1975) for the World Health Organization.

Emotional Disturbance—depression, hallucinations, distortions of reality, fantasies, "nervous breakdown," problems with "nerves," anxiety, excessive use of alcohol and other mind-altering drugs, suicidal and other self-destructive acts.

Hyperactive Behavior—inappropriate overactivity; wild, difficult to handle behavior.

Aggressive Conduct Disorder—fighting, bullying, destructive behavior, unsocialized aggression, temper tantrums, impulsive behavior, sexual aggression, assault.

Antisocial Behavior—delinquent and illegal acts, including theft, arson, inappropriate nonaggressive sexual behavior, refusal to attend school, excessive driving offenses, running away, and other violations of the law not defined as aggressive conduct disorder.

We employed a five-point scale of severity, 1 indicating mild behavior disturbance, and 5 severe behavior disturbance. No evidence of behavior disturbance was given a score of zero. For each person in the study, the rating on each of these four components of behavior disturbance was based on the amount of time and the degree to which the problem impaired that person's ability to function in expected activities. Also taken into account was evidence of concern about the behavior by the individuals themselves, their families, or local authorities, a definition influenced by Rutter, Tizard, and Whitmore (1970). The four types did not always occur singly, and when more than one was present, a rating was made for each.

Overall Behavior Disturbance

The rating scale used for each type of behavior disturbance was also used to obtain an overall rating that considered all the evidence of behavior disturbance for each person. The behavior ratings were made for two age periods: childhood up to age 15, and the age span of 16 to 22 years. The overall rating was never less severe than the rating for the most severe of the four types, but it could be more severe.

The evidence used in evaluating behavior disturbance was obtained from the interviews with the young people and the parents, and from agency records. For some young people in long-term services, the service providers who knew them well provided information.

This chapter differs from our previously published papers on behavior disturbance (Koller et al. 1982, 1983; Richardson, Koller, and Katz 1985a,b) in some ways. In order to compare the follow-up study with previous studies using the dichotomy of present and absent, and to simplify reporting, we will consider a rating of moderate to severe (3–5 on the scale) as indicating the presence of behavior disturbance, and a rating of none, mild, and mild-moderate (0–2 on the scale) as indicating the absence of behavior disturbance. Moderate to severe ratings reflect a degree of behavior disturbance sufficient to bring it to the attention of the various local authorities with professional concerns in this area. In the papers by Koller et al. and by Richardson, Koller, and Katz, the full six-point scale was used. These publications also provide statistical analyses as well as a full description of the methods used in evaluating evidence of behavior disturbance and reliability tests of the ratings. Reliability was excellent. Here, we give descriptive results.

Behavior Disturbance among Those with MR and Comparisons

The young people with MR, both males and females, had overall behavior disturbance and all four types at each age period more frequently than the comparisons (see Table 8.1). Most of these differences were statistically significant, but there was wide variation in the size of the differences. For males, the largest differences emerged in aggressive conduct disorder in childhood; for females, in emotional disturbance and aggressive conduct disorder. For males, a large difference occurred in antisocial behavior in childhood and diminished

Table 8.1 Frequency of moderate to severe behavior disturbance (overall and types) for those with MR and comparisons by gender in childhood and young adulthood, in percent

Behavior disturbance	Status	Males (n = 96)[a]		Females (n = 77)[a]	
		Childhood	Adulthood	Childhood	Adulthood
Overall	MR	39	34	35	42
	Comparison	6	15	3	5
Emotional	MR	11	14	23	30
	Comparison	4	3	0	4
Aggressive conduct	MR	22	18	17	20
	Comparison	1	6	1	1
Antisocial	MR	21	21	4	6
	Comparison	4	11	1	0
Hyperactivity	MR	7	2	5	1
	Comparison	1	0	0	0

a. n is the number of matched pairs of those with and without MR.

somewhat in the young adult period due to an increase in antisocial behavior among the comparisons. For females, the smallest difference was for antisocial behavior in childhood due to the low frequencies of this type of behavior.

Behavior Disturbance among the Young People with MR

Overall Behavior Disturbance in the Two Age Periods

Table 8.2 shows that the amount of behavior disturbance in the total population of young people with MR was virtually the same in the two age periods of childhood (37 percent) and young adulthood (38 percent). When males and females were examined separately, there was a slight decrease for males from childhood (39 percent) to adulthood (34 percent), whereas for the females there was some increase (35 percent and 42 percent, respectively). These increases and decreases were present in all four of the IQ categories—below 50, 50–59, 60–69, and 70 and above—for both males and females, with the one exception of males with IQ's of 60 to 69, where there was no change. At both age periods the highest frequency of behavior disturbance was found among those, both males and females, with IQ's of 70 and above.

Types of Behavior Disturbance

Two types of behavior disturbance showed a gender difference: more emotional disturbance was found among females and more antisocial behavior found among males (see Table 8.2), and these differences were statistically significant. Emotional disturbance was twice as frequent among females as males for all IQ groups combined, and females had consistently higher frequencies at each IQ level and in both age periods. For females, the amount of emotional disturbance was higher in adulthood than childhood at all IQ levels except 60 to 69, where there was no change. Young people with IQ's below 50 had less emotional disturbance than those with IQ's of 50 and above (although this may be due to the difficulty in diagnosing emotional disturbance in those with severe MR because of severely impaired communication). This finding held for males and females at both age periods, with the one exception of adult females, where those

Table 8.2 Frequency of moderate to severe behavior disturbance by IQ group and sex for childhood and adulthood

	Males (n = 111)									
	IQ <50 (n = 20)		IQ 50–59 (n = 25)		IQ 60–69 (n = 35)		IQ 70+ (n = 31)		Total	
Moderate to severe behavior disturbance	*N*	(%)	*N*	(%)	*N*	(%)	*N*	(%)	*N*	(%)
Overall										
Childhood	8	(40)	8	(32)	12	(35)	15	(48)	43	(39)
Adulthood	5	(25)	7	(28)	12	(35)	14	(45)	38	(34)
Emotional										
Childhood	1	(5)	3	(12)	2	(6)	6	(19)	12	(11)
Adulthood	1	(5)	4	(16)	5	(14)	5	(16)	15	(14)
Aggressive Conduct										
Childhood	7	(35)	6	(24)	5	(14)	6	(19)	24	(22)
Adulthood	4	(20)	2	(8)	9	(26)	5	(16)	20	(18)
Antisocial										
Childhood	1	(5)	4	(16)	9	(26)	9	(29)	23	(21)
Adulthood	1	(5)	4	(16)	9	(26)	9	(29)	23	(21)
Hyperactivity										
Childhood	5	(25)	2	(8)	1	(3)	0		8	(7)
Adulthood	1	(5)	1	(4)	0		0		2	(2)

	Females (n = 81)									
	IQ <50 (n = 16)		IQ 50–59 (n = 20)		IQ 60–69 (n = 34)		IQ 70+ (n = 11)		Total	
	N	(%)	*N*	(%)	*N*	(%)	*N*	(%)	*N*	(%)
Overall										
Childhood	6	(38)	7	(35)	10	(29)	5	(45)	28	(35)
Adulthood	7	(44)	8	(40)	13	(38)	6	(55)	34	(42)
Emotional										
Childhood	2	(13)	5	(25)	9	(26)	3	(27)	19	(23)
Adulthood	4	(25)	6	(30)	9	(26)	5	(45)	24	(30)
Aggressive Conduct										
Childhood	6	(38)	2	(10)	4	(13)	2	(18)	14	(17)
Adulthood	4	(25)	5	(25)	6	(18)	1	(9)	16	(20)
Antisocial										
Childhood	0		0		1	(3)	2	(18)	3	(4)
Adulthood	0		1	(5)	3	(9)	1	(9)	5	(6)
Hyperactivity										
Childhood	3	(19)	1	(5)	1	(3)	0		4	(5)
Adulthood	1	(6)	0		0		0		1	(1)

with IQ's below 50 had the same amount of emotional disturbance as those with IQ's of 60 to 69.

Antisocial behavior was three to five times more frequent among males than females, for whom it was rare, and the amount was virtually the same in the two age periods. Among males, the frequency of antisocial behavior increased as IQ increased; among females, what little antisocial behavior there was, was limited mainly to those with IQ's of 60 and above.There were no clear gender differences in aggressive conduct disorder. The highest frequency of aggressive conduct disorder was found among children of both sexes with IQ below 50, and this decreased for them as young adults. Hyperactivity was the least common of the four types of behavior disturbance. In childhood, it was most frequent among those, both males and females, with IQ's below 50. In adulthood, hyperactivity was rare, and it was absent among those with IQ's of 60 and above. Hyperactivity was more frequent among males than females.

Behavior Disturbance in Childhood as a Risk Factor

The preceding sections have examined behavior disturbance separately for the two age periods, and group differences in the two periods. In this section, we will examine whether behavior remained the same for each individual or changed as he or she grew from childhood into young adulthood.

One half of the population of young people with MR had no behavior disturbance in either of the age periods, and one quarter had behavior disturbance in both periods (see Table 8.3). The two smallest groups had behavior disturbance for only one period. Children

Table 8.3 Continuity and change in overall behavior disturbance between childhood and adulthood for MR study population

Behavior disturbance in childhood	Behavior disturbance in young adulthood		
	No	Yes	Total
No	95	26	121
Yes	25	46	71
Total	120	72	192

with behavior disturbance were at far higher risk of continued behavior disturbance as young adults than children who did not. Sixty-five percent (46/71) of the children who had behavior disturbance continued to have behavior disturbance as young adults, compared to only 21 percent (26/121) of those who did not have behavior disturbance as children.

The risk of adult behavior disturbance may vary, depending on the type of disturbance the adult experienced as a child. To examine this possibility, we organized the four types of behavioral disturbance as follows in order to compare our findings with those of Rutter et al. (1977):

Conduct Disorder—aggressive conduct disorder and/or antisocial behavior.
Emotional Disorder—the category was retained intact when it was the only type of disorder for an individual.
Mixed Behavior Disturbance—conduct disorder in combination with emotional disturbance or hyperactivity.

For both males and females, children with conduct disorders had more adult behavior disturbance than those with emotional or mixed disorders (see Table 8.4). This agrees with the findings of Rutter and his colleagues. The worst prognosis was for girls with conduct disorders, where 100 percent continued with behavior disturbance as young adults. The best prognosis was for boys with emotional disturbance, where only 29 percent continued to have behavior disturbance.

The chronicity involved in the continuation of conduct disorders

Table 8.4 Children with emotional, conduct, and mixed disorders who, as young adults, did and did not have moderate to severe overall behavior disturbance

Gender	Period(s) with behavior disturbance	Emotional	Conduct	Mixed
Males	Childhood only	5	6	4
	Childhood and adulthood	2	19	6
Females	Childhood only	4	0	5
	Childhood and adulthood	8	7	4

from childhood to the young adult years can best be illustrated by examining two case histories.[2]

One boy was taken away from his mother and stepfather at age 12, after persistent truancy and delinquency, and committed to the care of the city authorities. As early as age 7, he had been described in school records as destructive, aggressive, and untruthful. At age 15 he was sent to an Approved (Reform) School; after eighteen months he was transferred to a Borstal (a penal residence for juvenile delinquents) and released a year later. Following that, he had a record of about 20 arrests for various crimes, mainly theft, but also housebreaking, reckless discharge of a firearm, resisting arrest, and driving with a revoked license. He was sentenced four times to institutions for youthful offenders for periods ranging from one to nine months. According to our records, his last court appearance was a few months prior to our interview with him at age 22.

Another boy began getting into trouble at age 9, and he, too, was eventually removed from his parents' home. Between ages 11 and 20, he appeared in court twenty-one times, with ten charges of theft, thirteen of breaking and entering, one of vandalism; six breaches of the peace, seven driving offenses, and one charge of fraud. He had stolen from his parents, beaten his mother, and was evicted for using his house as a brothel. At 22, he was under an eight-year driving ban after knocking down a policeman.

Other case histories may help to illustrate the recovery from childhood emotional disturbance in the young adult years. Most were from moderate emotional disturbance, but one young woman recovered from severe emotional disturbance. Her mother reported that an incident when she was six years old had caused her emotional problems. There was a fire at a neighbor's house, which she witnessed, with policemen and firemen running up and down, and her father going in to help. Her mother reported that the child screamed for a long while, and a great fear set in, causing her speech to regress and

2. As we noted in the Preface, the largely quantitative presentation of our results is intended to protect the anonymity of individuals. When we illustrate some of the findings with brief case histories, we have changed any identifying information while maintaining the features that illustrate the particular point we are making. We are deeply grateful to the study population and their parents who told us so much about themselves and have been vigilant in safeguarding the data we collected as well as those we obtained from other research sources.

an eye to turn in. She was extremely fearful for a long time after the incident, but she seemed to do well after leaving school.

Two other girls had similar histories of moderate emotional disturbance in early childhood. They were both described as weepy, tense, and frightened, and had sleeping problems. They were given sedative medication and both responded well. As the school years progressed, they required less and less sedation, and finally, between ages 10 and 12, they no longer needed it.

Factors Contributing to Behavior Disturbance

Our review of the literature suggested that four factors contribute to behavior disturbance. The first was brain dysfunction. To examine whether brain dysfunction contributed to behavior disturbance, we used the clinical judgments of Dr. Keith Goulden, a pediatric neurologist, which he based on the medical history of the child and the mother's reproductive history. The evidence was ordered according to the probability that there were indicators of brain dysfunction. They included genetic abnormalities, cerebral malformations, postnatal injuries, cerebral palsy, microcephaly, macrocephaly, uncomplicated epilepsy, autism, and being small for gestational age (Richardson et al. 1990). We found no significant difference in the amount of behavior disturbance in childhood or young adulthood among those with different levels of probability of brain dysfunction. These results provide no evidence that brain dysfunction was a contributing factor to behavior disturbance.

Epilepsy is a manifestation of brain dysfunction, and behavior disturbance has been found to be more common among people with epilepsy than among the general population (Rutter, Tizard, and Whitmore 1970; Dodrill and Batzel 1986; Whitman and Hermann 1986; Ounsted, Lindsay, and Richards 1987). As we report in Chapter 9, we looked for differences in the study population between those with and those without epilepsy but found none. This agreed with the findings of Goulden and Shinnar for a clinic population of children with developmental disabilities.

The other three possible explanations for behavior disturbance—psychosocial adversity, the dynamic of stress in a child with MR and in the family, which, in turn, causes behavior disturbance in the child, and the role of MR in increasing an individual's vulnerability to stress—all have stress as a common factor. The first two deal with stress that can affect the person, and the third with how the person copes with stress.

In Chapter 6, we used a family stability measure, with a five-point scale ranging from a stable to a highly unstable family environment during the child's upbringing, as an indicator of psychosocial adversity. If psychosocial adversity contributes to behavior disturbance, then increasingly unstable family environments should result in a corresponding increase in behavior disturbance. Table 8.5 shows that for children with MR, there was a steady increase in the amount of overall behavior disturbance as the amount of family instability increased. As young adults, the same increase occurred from 1 to 3 on the scale of family stability and then plateaued. At both age levels, the largest increase in behavior disturbance occurred between 2 and 3 on the scale.

There is no reason to believe that the relationship between family stability and behavior disturbance should be unique to those with MR, so we examined the same relationship for the nonretarded comparisons (see Table 8.5). Since only two of the comparisons experienced family instability of 4 or 5 on the scale, only 1 to 3 could be used to examine the relationship between family instability and behavior disturbance. But even for this restricted range, with increasing

Table 8.5 Percentages with moderate to severe behavior disturbance in childhood and as young adults by family stability for young people with mental retardation and comparisons

	Family stability				
	Stable 1	2	3	4	Unstable 5
All children with MR	23%	30%	49%	50%	59%
All comparison children	2%	5%	12.5%		
All young adults with MR	18%	28%	61.5%	57%	55.5%
All comparison young adults	1%	3%	25%		
Total with MR	65	47	39	14	27
Total comparisons	103	59	8		

family instability there was also an increasing amount of behavior disturbance in both childhood and young adulthood, with a major increase between 2 and 3.

If family instability were the only factor contributing to behavior disturbance, the same rates of behavior disturbance would be found among those with and those without mental retardation when controlling for level of family stability. As Table 8.5 shows, at each point on the scale, the young people with mental retardation showed markedly more behavior disturbance. This suggests there were additional factors contributing to behavior disturbance among those with MR that were not present among the comparisons. Tarjan (1977), as we have noted, suggested one such factor: individuals with MR are highly vulnerable to emotional trauma.

The suggestion that a child with MR causes stress on the family, and this, in turn, causes behavior disturbance in the child, could not be directly tested from our data. This sequence of events is most plausible under conditions in which a child has severe MR as well as additional disabilities, such as epilepsy or cerebral palsy. These circumstances were present for only a small number of the children in the study. The degree of intellectual impairment alone among the children with mild MR would not have placed a heavy burden of care on the family. The stress of having a child with mild MR may be greater, as suggested by Farber (1968), for families at the upper end of the socioeconomic scale or families concerned with upward social mobility. In our study, for 92 percent of the children with mild MR, the head of the family was a manual worker, and a considerable number of families lived in conditions that have been described in the mental retardation literature as contributing to sociocultural retardation. In such a family, a child with mild MR might not be regarded as deviant and thus might not be a source of stress.

Those with MR experience additional forms of stress, either uniquely or more often, than nonretarded people. Concern that classifying a child as MR has stigmatizing consequences for the child has been growing (see Chapter 5 for a discussion of this question). To the extent that this occurs, it is a form of stress unique to the children so classified. We have already shown that children with MR experienced more family instability than the nonretarded comparisons. In addition, even when stable, the families of children with mild MR may experience more of other forms of stress resulting from low income and social incompetence. In the earlier study (see Chapter 1), Birch et al. (1970) found that the families of children with mild MR in the two lowest social classes were overrepresented within their social classes in living in undesirable neighborhoods, having more than five children, and having housing with a high person-to-room ratio.

We found that, as young adults, those with mild MR had lower incomes and poorer working conditions than the nonretarded comparisons (see Chapter 16). These conditions may more often be a source of stress for those with MR than for nonretarded comparisons. At various points in this book, we discuss other problems resulting from having MR, such as difficulties in literacy, numeracy, verbal communication, and social interactions, both during childhood and as young adults. Coping with these difficulties in everyday life is likely to impose unique stresses.It is clear that the sources of stress for individuals with MR in general are many, and probably greater, than those experienced by people without MR.

Other intrinsic factors include brain dysfunction, for which we found no relationship with behavior disturbance. The only other intrinsic factor we could examine was that of intergenerational genetic disorders, which we have called Family Pedigree (see Chapter 6). We examined the relationship between Family Pedigree and behavior disturbance in both periods, and its relationship to behavior disturbance in the context of family stability, using a multiple regression analysis. In both of these analyses, Family Pedigree showed no relationship to behavior disturbance.

Comparisons with Previous Research

The follow-up study agrees with previous research that behavior disturbance is more common among those with MR than those without MR. Of the four types of behavior disturbance examined, antisocial behavior has been the major focus of previous research. For methodological reasons, earlier results need to be accepted with caution, but a higher rate of antisocial behavior among those with MR was indicated, and our results agreed. Among males, we found that antisocial behavior in childhood was more common among those with MR. In adulthood, however, the difference diminished somewhat because of an increase in antisocial behavior among young adults without MR.

Of the children with severe MR, 39 percent were found to have behavior disturbance, a rate close to the median rate of the previous studies we reviewed. For the age period of 16 to 22, however, there were no previous studies of behavior disturbance among people with severe MR. We did not find a difference between the children with mild MR and severe MR in the amount of overall behavior disturbance, but two previous studies showed a slightly higher rate of behavior disturbance among children with severe MR (Birch et al. 1970; Gillberg et al. 1986). We found that somewhat more males with MR than females with MR had behavior disturbance in childhood, but we found the opposite in young adulthood. Previous studies of children found no clear gender differences.

9

Epilepsy

There have been many studies of epilepsy among individuals with mental retardation (MR) in institutions and among those seen in diagnostic and treatment centers on an outpatient basis. Yet, although these studies have made valuable contributions to our knowledge of epilepsy, they are inappropriate for determining its frequency and distribution in populations with mental retardation. Institutions and clinics see only selected samples of people, who are not representative of all those with mental retardation. Recently, however, a few epidemiological studies of epilepsy in representative populations of young people with mental retardation have been carried out. It has been observed for over a century that epilepsy is found more frequently among those with severe MR than among those with mild MR (Gower 1881). Investigators have therefore reported results separately for these two groups.

Epidemiological studies of epilepsy among young people with severe MR are summarized in Table 9.1. The prevalence of severe MR in these studies ranges from 2.6 per 1000 to 4.2 per 1000. These prevalence rates are close to those reviewed earlier (see Chapter 5) and suggest that the study populations are representative. The percentages of individuals with severe MR who also had epilepsy range from 18 percent to 40 percent, with a median of 28.5 percent.

Epidemiological studies of epilepsy among young people with mild MR are summarized in Table 9.2. The prevalence rates for mild MR

Table 9.1 Summary of prevalence and percentage of epilepsy among young people with severe mental retardation (IQ <50)

	Prevalence			
Study	Ages	Rate/1000 for severe MR	Place	Percentage with epilepsy
Shepherd and Hosking 1989	5–16	2.6	Sheffield, England	40
Gustavson et al. 1977a	6–16	3.9	Västerbotten, Sweden	36
Corbett 1983	0–14	3.9	Camberwell, England	33
Gustavson et al 1977b	5–16	2.8	Uppsala County, Sweden	30
Gillberg et al. 1986, 1983	13–17	3.5	Gothenberg, Sweden	27
McQueen et al. 1987	7–10	(IQ <55) 3.7	Canadian Maritime Prov.	23
Wald et al. 1977	15–24 (follow-up)	3.4	Poland	22
Cooper et al. 1979	7–16	4.2	Mannheim, Germany	18

range from 3.8 per 1000 to 7.5 per 1000, and are in line with the lower prevalence rates found in studies conducted in the 1980s. The percentages of those with mild MR and epilepsy range from 8.5 percent to 12 percent, with a median of 9.5 percent.

These studies clearly show that children with severe MR have about a three times greater risk of epilepsy than children with mild MR. In the general population, the frequency of epilepsy is far lower than that found even for mild MR. Corbett, Harris, and Robinson (1975), in a review of several studies, estimated the frequency of epilepsy in the general population of schoolchildren as 0.7 percent.

Previous studies show that, in addition to severity of mental retardation, there are other factors that alter the degree of risk of developing epilepsy. In the Camberwell study of children with severe MR, seizures occurred in 60 percent of children who also had cerebral palsy, but in only 20 percent of those without cerebral palsy (Corbett 1981). Shepherd and Hosking (1989) subdivided children with mild MR and severe MR into groups with and without a "physical disability." Among those with mild MR and no physical disability, 7 percent had epilepsy, compared with 41 percent among those with a physical disability. Among children with severe MR and no physical disability, 26 percent had epilepsy, compared with 67 percent among those with a physical disability. Benedetti et al. (1986) and Hauser et al. (1987)

Table 9.2 Summary of prevalence and percentage of epilepsy among young children with mild mental retardation (IQ 50–69)

	Prevalence			
Study	Ages	Rate/1000 for mild MR	Place	Percentage with epilepsy
Shepherd and Hosking 1989	5–16	6.3	Sheffield, England	9
Gillberg et al. 1983, 1986	13–17	5.6	Gothenberg, Sweden	10
Blomquist et al. 1981	8–19	3.8	Swedish county	12
Hagberg et al. 1981b	8–12	4.0	Gothenberg, Sweden	12
Lamont and Dennis 1988	7–11	7.5	Southampton, England	8.5

have shown, in a clinic-based population of severely disabled children, that the risk of epilepsy was 11 percent for those with mental retardation alone and 48 percent for those with mental retardation and cerebral palsy. Studies of children with cerebral palsy report a much higher incidence of seizures when mental retardation is present (Lagergren 1981). Cerebral palsy is, therefore, a reasonable marker for underlying brain injury that has also led to MR and epilepsy.

Other markers of underlying brain injury may also be associated with an increased risk for epilepsy. There is evidence, for example, that head trauma increases the risk of epilepsy (Annegers et al. 1980; Salazar et al. 1985). In a study of children with severe MR, Wald (1977) subdivided those with epilepsy according to different categories of etiology of mental retardation and found that epilepsy occurred most frequently in categories of postnatal factors (infections, poisoning, and injury).

Epilepsy may occur at different ages. The risk of developing epilepsy among individuals with MR is not restricted to early childhood but exists as well during the school years and into early adulthood (Benedetti et al. 1986; Hauser et al. 1987). In terms of remission, it is well known that in general populations, individuals with epilepsy can enter remission (Hauser and Kurland 1975; Annegers, Hauser, and Elveback 1979a). Favorable factors for remission include childhood onset and normal neurological status; unfavorable factors include the presence of a neurological handicap, particularly if it is congenital. In their study in Rochester, Minnesota, Hauser and Kurland (1975) found that 70 percent of those with childhood onset of idiopathic epilepsy were in remission (defined as five years without seizures, with or without medication) twenty years after the diagnosis. In the group with mental retardation or cerebral palsy and epilepsy, however, only 40 percent were in remission twenty years after the onset of their seizure disorders.

A separate issue, which has been of considerable interest, is whether people with epilepsy are at greater risk of having behavior disturbance than people without epilepsy. This has been found to be so in general populations (Rutter, Graham, and Yule 1970; Dodrill and Batzell 1986; Whitman and Hermann 1986; Ounsted, Lindsay, and Richards 1987), but less attention has been paid to this issue among populations with MR. Goulden and Shinnar (1989) examined this issue in a clinic for children with developmental disabilities, selecting for study those with both MR and cerebral palsy. They concluded that epilepsy was not an additional risk factor for behavior disturbance.

This review provides the context for the analysis of our study population, which examines the risk of epilepsy over the first twenty-two years of life, dividing the cohort by markers of underlying brain injury.

To identify epilepsy in our follow-up study population, we used multiple sources of evidence covering their twenty-two years of life. We obtained some information from the life history interview with the parents of each subject. Parents were asked, "Did your child ever have fits?" (the term used locally). If their response was yes, we inquired further about the age when the seizures started and ended, the type and frequency of the seizures, any use of anticonvulsant drugs, and any side effects of the drugs.

We also examined a number of documentary sources for evidence of seizures, including the records kept by the health visitors, who were required by statute to visit all children at home during their early years; school medical records; reports of the social work department; records of the mental retardation services; a pediatric neurological examination given to three of the five birth cohorts in the earlier study when the children were 8 to 10 years of age; and data from a regional mental retardation survey of the northeast of Scotland carried out shortly before our study (Innes, Johnston, and Millar 1978).

In addition, Dr. Keith Goulden, a member of our research team, examined the cumulative hospital records for everyone in the study, including electroencephalogram (EEG) records kept for many years by the regional EEG laboratory. All information relating to seizures was collated for each person and reviewed by two pediatric neurologists. Epilepsy was defined as "clear evidence of recurrent unprovoked seizures." The final classification of epilepsy was made by Dr. Goulden and Dr. Shlomo Shinnar. Of the 221 young people with MR in the cohort, the data were sufficient to determine seizures histories for all but 4.

The Four Groups

The study population was divided into three clinical subtypes and a fourth miscellaneous group (Goulden et al. 1992):

Mental Retardation Only. Young people who had no motor handicap, and whose mental retardation was of known prenatal or perinatal origin, or of unknown origin ($n = 152$).

Mental Retardation and Cerebral Palsy (CP). Individuals with MR and CP whose developmental disabilities were of known or presumed prenatal or perinatal origin ($n = 32$).

Postnatal Injury (PNI). Individuals with a history of postnatal brain injury sufficient to have caused mental retardation ($n = 15$), including four with motor disfunction *resulting from* postnatal injury, and 11 with "symptomatic" seizures (present at the time of onset of injury).

Genetic and Other. Miscellaneous group consisting of individuals with autosomal, sex chromosome, and single gene disorders, and one person with a cerebral malformation ($n = 18$).

Summary Disability Scale

For our broader research purposes, we needed a measure of the degree to which having epilepsy interfered with an individual's usual daily activities. We used the following variables: proportion of time within the stage of life (defined below) when there were seizures; frequency of seizures within that time; severity of symptoms; use of anticonvulsant medication; and side effects of medication. These five variables were combined into a classification with four degrees of disability, which was applied to four stages of development: preschool (0–5 years); early school (6–11 years); late school (12–15 years), and postschool (16–22 years). (The details of the classification and its application at each stage for all seizure cases can be found in Richardson et al. 1981. A summary classification of degree of disability was then developed that spanned the entire history from birth to age 22.

Table 9.3 provides comparative data from our follow-up study: there were 33 cases of epilepsy among the 217 young people with mental retardation (15 percent). For those with severe MR (IQ <50), the frequency was 35 percent, and for those with mild MR (IQ 50+), it was 10 percent (17/171). The other studies shown in Table 9.2 defined mild MR as IQ 50–69. When we use the same IQ range, 12 percent (15/124) had epilepsy, the top end of the range shown in Table 9.2.

On the basis of previous research, we anticipated that those in the cerebral palsy (CP) and postnatal injury (PNI) subtypes would have higher rates of epilepsy than those with mental retardation only, and Table 9.3 (line e) shows that the frequencies of epilepsy in the three subtypes were strikingly different: MR alone, 5 percent; CP, 38 percent; and PNI, 73 percent. In the fourth group, a heterogeneous mix of people, the rate was 11 percent.

For the subtype with PNI, which showed the highest rate of epilepsy, the percentage of those with epilepsy increased with the severity of mental retardation (Table 9.3, lines a and d). By contrast, for the

Table 9.3 Percentage with epilepsy in the four groups and IQ distribution of each subtype

	MR alone		MR and cerebral palsy		MR and postnatal injury		MR and genetic and other		Total	
IQ	*N*	(%)	*N*	(%)	*N*	(%)	*N*	(%)	*N*	(%)
a. <50	0/13	(0)	7/14	(50)	7/7	(100)	2/12	(17)	16/46	(35)
b. 50–59	2/35	(6)	4/4	(100)	2/3	(67)	0/4	(0)	8/46	(17)
c. 60–69	4/62	(6)	1/10	(10)	2/4	(50)	0/2	(0)	7/78	(9)
d. 70+	2/42	(5)	0/4	(0)	0/1	(0)	0/0	(0)	2/47	(4)
e. Total with epilepsy	8/152	(5)	12/32	(38)	11/15	(73)	2/18	(11)	33/217	(15)

subtype with MR alone, there was no one with both epilepsy and severe MR, and the percentage with epilepsy did not vary across the subdivisions of IQ in the mild MR range. However, even when IQ was controlled for at both IQ levels between 50 and 70, there was a higher percentage with epilepsy in the subtypes with CP and PNI than in the subtype with MR alone. (In this population, there were only 13 children with severe MR and no other disabilities, so the confidence intervals for estimates of epilepsy in this group are quite large.)

At each IQ level from IQ 70+ to IQ <50, the percentage with epilepsy for the total population doubled. This increase in percentage as IQ decreased is clearly related to the clinical subtypes, CP and PNI making the greatest contribution to the relationship.

To determine the degree of overall disability found as a consequence of epilepsy, we used the summary disability scale described above. Table 9.4 shows that 14/30 (47 percent) of all persons with epilepsy were severely or moderately severely disabled by it. The subtypes with CP and PNI included a higher proportion who were severely or moderately severely disabled than the subtype with MR alone. Those in the subtype with PNI were the most disabled of all.

Twenty individuals had seizures initially considered to be febrile convulsions. These were defined as seizures accompanied by fever after one month of age, not associated with an acute neurological illness or electrolyte imbalance, in children with no prior history of

Table 9.4 Severity of disability resulting from epilepsy by group

	MR alone		MR and cerebral palsy		MR and postnatal injury		MR and genetic and other		Total	
	N	(%)	*N*	(%)	*N*	(%)	*N*	(%)	*N*	(%)
Severe (5)	0		3	(25)	2	(20)	1	(50)	6	(20)
Moderate severe (4)	2	(25)	3	(25)	5	(50)	0		8	(27)
Moderate (3)	4	(50)	5[a]	(42)	2	(20)	1	(50)	12	(40)
Mild (2)	2	(25)	1	(8)	1	(10)	0		4	(13)
Total	8		12		10[b]		2		30	

a. For 2 of the cases classified as moderate, there was an inadequate history to make a classification with confidence. The classification of these cases is conservative, based on available data.

b. An additional child died at age 9, so no summary classification can be made over the twenty-two year period. Epilepsy was severe over his lifetime.

afebrile seizures (Hauser and Kurland 1975; Nelson and Ellenberg 1976). Seven of the twenty (35 percent) went on to develop epilepsy. The remaining 13 experienced febrile seizures only. In the subtypes with MR alone, and with MR and CP, children with and without febrile seizures had a similar risk of developing epilepsy.

Epilepsy at Different Ages

By following the study population up to age 22 we were able to examine the ages when epilepsy first occurred, when remissions took place, and the duration of the epilepsy in the population as a whole and for the three discrete clinical subtypes.

We first examined the cumulative probability of developing epilepsy up to age 22. The cumulative probability is computed as the product of the proportion of individuals with epilepsy at age 22 and the proportion with epilepsy in all previous one-year periods. This computation assumes a common starting point for all cases, but this does not occur for all the young people with epilepsy. For the subtypes with MR only and with MR and CP, it was considered that the risk of both mental retardation and epilepsy began at birth. For the subtype with PNI, however, the risk of MR and epilepsy began only at the time of the PNI. To take this difference in timing into account, Kaplan-Meier methodology was used (Kaplan and Meier 1958). The same form of analysis was used in calculating remission rates. The significance of the difference between remission curves was calculated nonparametrically using Peto and Peto's (1972) generalized Wilcoxen test.

The cumulative risk of developing epilepsy for all the young people with mental retardation is shown in Figure 9.1. The incremental rate was greatest in the first two to three years of life, but new cases of epilepsy continued to occur up to age 20. Figure 9.2 shows the cumulative probability for the three clinical subtypes. The fourth group was included in the overall analysis but omitted from the subtype analyses because of its heterogeneity. The incremental rate was greater at earlier ages for the subtypes with MR and CP and with MR and PNI than for those with MR alone. There were no gender differences in the cumulative risk in any of the three subtypes.

We next examined rates of remission, defined as being seizure-free for five years, with or without medication (Hauser and Kurland

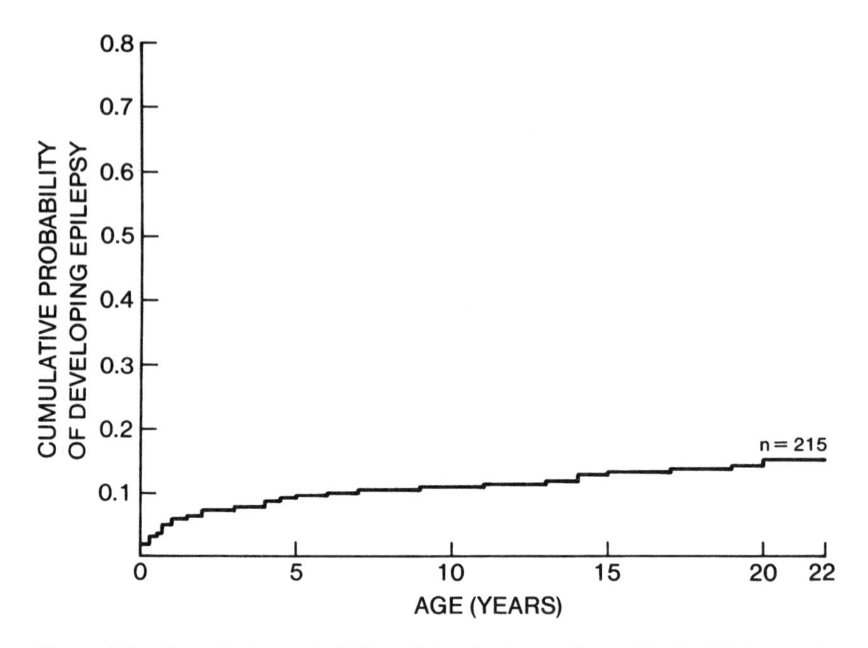

Figure 9.1 Cumulative probability of developing epilepsy, Kaplan-Meier analysis. Reprinted with permission from Goulden et al. 1992.

1975). Of the total group with epilepsy (n = 33), 39 percent had attained remission by age 22 (Figure 9.3). The rates of remission were 56 percent in the subtype with MR only, 47 percent in the subtype with MR and CP, and 11 percent in the subtype with MR and PNI (Figure 9.4). The Kaplan-Meier curves for remission in the first two subgroups are not significantly different from one another, but these subtypes both differed significantly from the subtype with PNI ($p < .05$).

Because of treatment patterns at the time of the study, most young people with seizures received anti-epileptic medication indefinitely. Four young people (three in the subtype with MR only and one in the subtype with PNI) were in five-year remission without medication. Of those not achieving five-year remission, 80 percent were still receiving medication at the time of follow-up at 22 years of age. It should be noted that 10 percent of the population had been or were still being treated with phenobarbital (for "behavioral problems") at follow-up, although they had no history of epilepsy. A detailed discussion of the actual treatment practices is outside the scope of this observational study and would not be helpful because of the changes in practice occurring over the last thirty years.

Ages When Epilepsy Was Present

The duration of time and the ages at which epilepsy was present for each person is shown in Figure 9.5, together with their clinical subtypes, gender, and IQ. Eleven people had epilepsy for twenty years or more, fourteen for six to nineteen years, and eight for five years or less. One died at age 9 after having had epilepsy for eight years. Those in the subtypes with MR and CP and with MR and PNI had epilepsy for a longer time than those with MR alone, and males for longer than females. Among those whose epilepsy lasted five years or

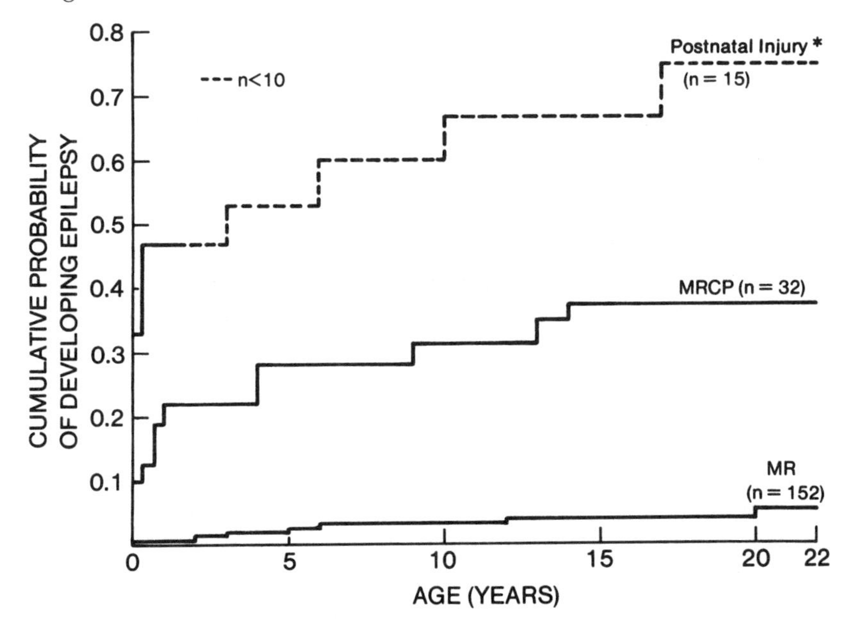

Figure 9.2 Cumulative probability of developing epilepsy in three subgroups: MR–mental retardation of presumed prenatal, perinatal, or unknown etiology, without associated disability, known genetic syndrome, or postnatal injury; MRCP–MR associated with cerebral palsy of presumed prenatal or perinatal etiology; Postnatal Injury–MR associated with postnatal injury. Risk for last group calculated from the time of injury. Kaplan-Meier analysis. Reprinted with permission from Goulden et al. 1992.

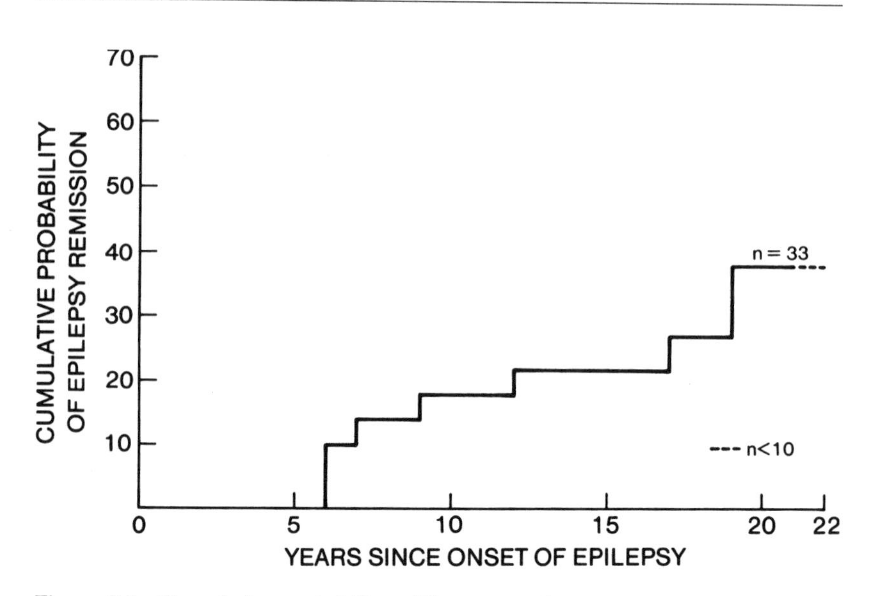

Figure 9.3 Cumulative probability of five-year epilepsy remission. Probabilities calculated from time of onset of epilepsy. Kaplan-Meier analysis. Dotted line indicates that <10 subjects with active epilepsy were still in follow-up. Reprinted with permission from Goulden et al. 1992.

less, there was no particular age span when the epilepsy was present more often. There was a positive relationship, however, between the duration of time an individual experienced the epilepsy and the severity of the disability due to epilepsy.

Behavior Disturbance and Epilepsy

As we noted earlier, behavior disturbance in the general population has been found to be more common among those with epilepsy than those without it. There has been less research on whether children with MR are at higher risk of behavior disturbance when they also have epilepsy. We examined the frequency and severity of overall behavior disturbance (see Chapter 8) among those with and without epilepsy for all those with MR and separately among those with mild MR and severe MR; we found no significant differences. This finding is in accord with that of Goulden et al. (1992) for children with developmental disorders.

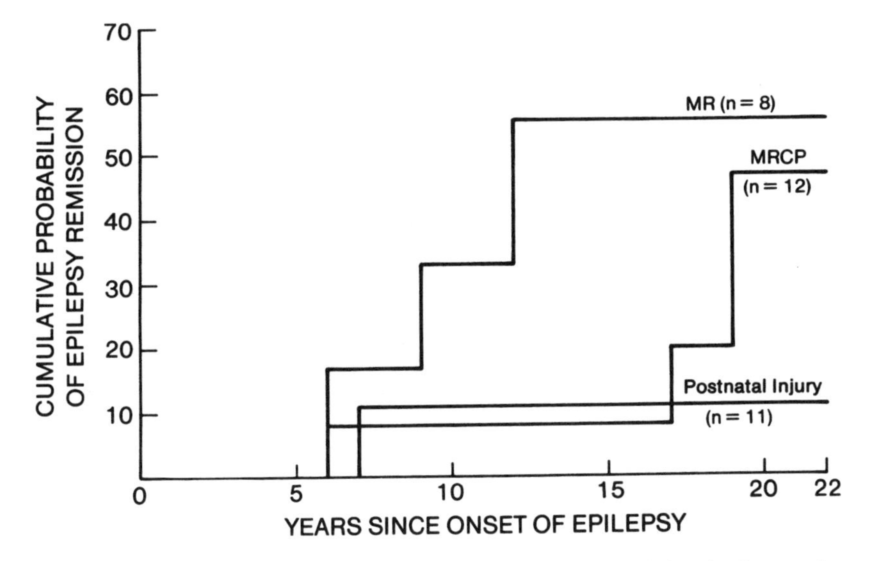

Figure 9.4 Cumulative probability of five-year epilepsy remission in three subgroups. Definitions of subgroups are as in Figure 9.2. Two cases from postnatal injury group excluded. Probabilities calculated from time of onset of epilepsy. Kaplan-Meier analysis. Reprinted with permission from Goulden et al. 1992.

The question "What percentage of those with mental retardation also have epilepsy?" is complex. The answer depends on the interplay of the definitions of mental retardation and epilepsy, the population at risk, age, and whether a cross-sectional or longitudinal view is adopted. For comparison, we selected epidemiological studies whose populations and definitions were similar to ours. In the studies of people with severe MR, the range with epilepsy was 18 percent to 40 percent, with a median of 28.5 percent; we found 36 percent, the same percentage obtained by Gustavson et al. (1977a) and similar to that found by Shepherd and Hosking (1989), who may have used a broader definition of epilepsy than we did. The 22-year lifespan used in our follow-up study would be expected to yield a higher percentage with epilepsy than studies that were cross-sectional or used a shorter follow-up period.

The rates of epilepsy given in previous studies of young people with mild MR show a surprisingly narrow range (9 percent to 12 percent). The 9 percent was obtained by Cooper et al. (1979), who included a 40 percent sample of children with borderline mental retardation

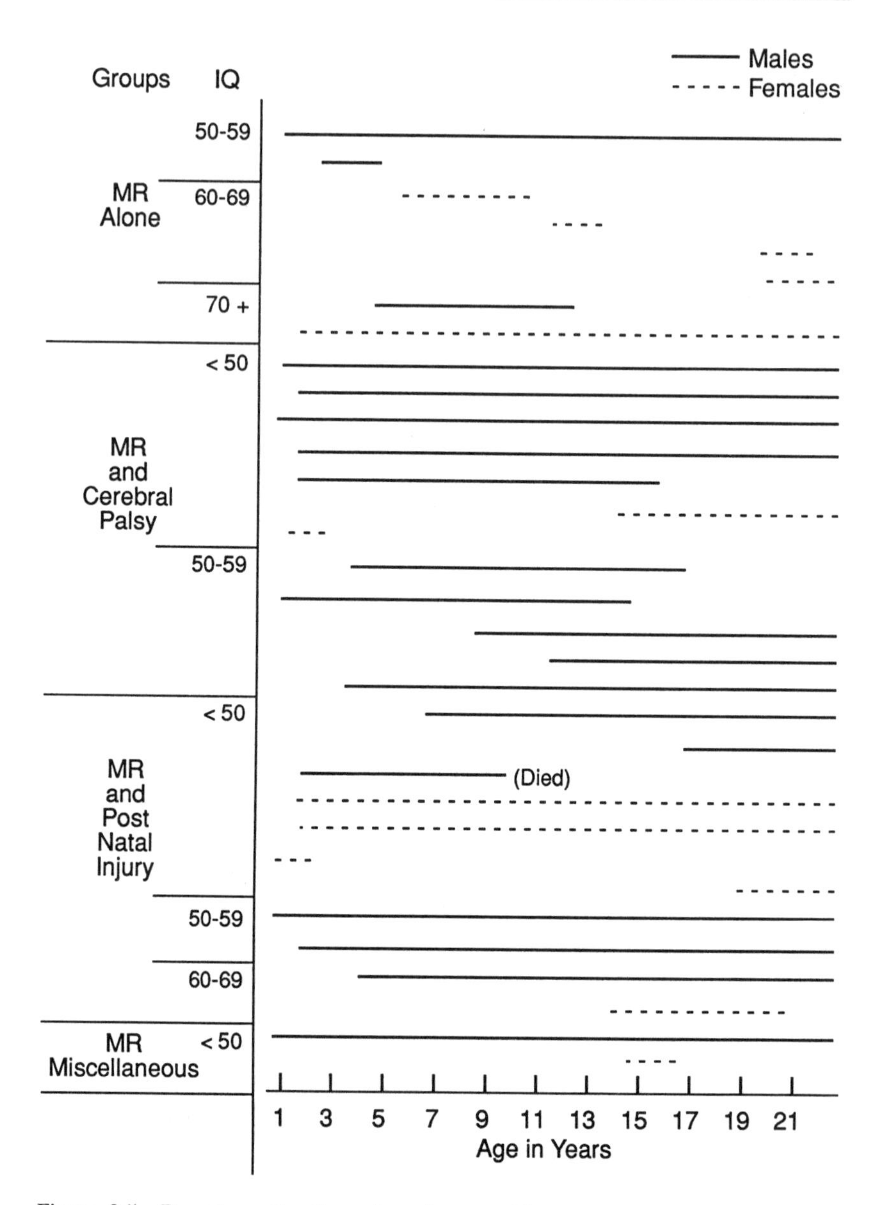

Figure 9.5 Duration of epilepsy by subgroup, IQ group, and gender.

(IQ 70+). When we used an upper IQ cut off point of 70 for the population with mild MR, we found 12 percent with epilepsy, which is very close to the previous results. Again, because the present study was conducted over a longer period of time than the other studies, a higher percentage of epilepsy might be expected.Our results are consonant with those of the studies we reviewed, which show that epilepsy occurs more frequently among individuals with severe MR than with mild MR, and that both groups have higher frequencies than the general population.

There were major differences in the risk of developing epilepsy, depending on the clinical subtype to which young people with MR belonged. The lowest risk (5 percent) was for those with MR only, higher than the approximately 0.7 percent for general populations of school children. By contrast, the risk of epilepsy was highest for those whose MR was due to postnatal injury (73 percent), an expected finding in view of previous studies (Annegers et al. 1980; Salazer et al. 1985; Wald et al. 1977). The 73 percent risk for those with PNI may be attributed to sustained postnatal injuries severe enough to cause mental retardation and more severe than those of the average trauma or meningitis victim. The 38 percent rate of epilepsy for those with MR and CP was higher than the rate for MR alone, and this was also expected in view of previous studies. Severity of mental retardation, clinical subtype, and epilepsy were interrelated. Those with MR alone, all of whom had IQ's of 50 and above, had the lowest risk of epilepsy. Approximately half of those in the subtypes with CP and PNI had IQ's below 50, but even after we controlled for IQ, they were still at greater risk of epilepsy.

The fourth group, those with known genetic syndromes and malformations, is heterogeneous in terms of clinical and etiological factors but they are sufficiently distinct from those in the subtype with MR alone to be separated from them. Two of eighteen (11 percent) in this group had epilepsy, and both also had severe MR.

The measure of disability attributable to epilepsy provided some indication of the extent to which parents or caretakers might have experienced additional concerns and demands as a function of the epilepsy. It was intended to provide information that would complement the available classifications of epilepsy, which were intended primarily for medical purposes. When the measure was applied, 47 percent of those with epilepsy were rated as severely or moderately severely disabled due to seizures. Those with CP and PNI experienced more disabling consequences than those with MR alone. The disabling consequences of epilepsy need to be considered in the context of an individual's total disabilities. When MR is severe and accompanied by other severe disabilities, epilepsy may have less effect on a person's daily life than when MR is mild and epilepsy is the only other disability.

In the general population, the risk of epilepsy following febrile seizures is 2 percent to 7 percent (Nelson and Ellenberg 1976; Annegers et al. 1979b, 1987). This risk is higher for those with "abnormal neurological status" before the onset of febrile seizures. In the follow-up study, of the twenty people who had febrile convulsions, seven (35 percent) went on to develop epilepsy, a number much higher than in the general population but consistent with other studies of children with developmental disabilities.

For almost half the young people in the study population, the onset of epilepsy occurred during the first two years of life. Of the remaining cases of epilepsy, the onset was spread across the age range from 3 to 22 years, and 12 percent did not develop epilepsy until age 17 or later. This finding is consistent with a study of handicapped children in New York (Benedetti et al. 1986; Hauser et al. 1987). Those in the clinical subtypes with CP and PNI experienced early onset more frequently than those with MR alone.

People with all kinds of epilepsy can enter remission (Hauser and Kurland 1975; Annegers, Hauser, and Elveback 1979a). In their Rochester, Minnesota, study Hauser and Kurland (1975) found that those with MR or CP and epilepsy had a remission rate of 46 percent twenty years after the onset of their seizure disorder. In our study, we were not able to follow for twenty years those whose onset occurred at older ages, so our remission rate would be expected to be slightly lower. However, because most remission occurs early in the course of the disease, it is unclear whether this is a substantial effect. Our remission rate was 39 percent for the total population, with the highest in the subtype with MR alone and the lowest in the subtype with PNI.

The number of study subjects with epilepsy ($n = 33$) was small, but the differences among the subtypes in the proportions with epilepsy were strong enough to overcome the problems due to small numbers, and the agreement with other studies gave us confidence that the differences were valid. Other findings, that, for example, the duration of epilepsy was longer for males than for females, may need further corroboration before they can be considered valid. Our findings on the degree of disability due to the epilepsy are, as far as we know, unique, and the effect of epilepsy on a person's life bears further consideration.

10

Verbal Communication

There is a fundamental relationship between mental retardation (MR) and verbal communication. Abbeduto (1991) states, "Spoken language is involved in most types of social interaction and in classroom instruction; thus problems in verbal communication will have negative effects on many facets of an individual's mental and behavioral functioning" (p. 91). It seemed essential, then, in our follow-up study, to take account of verbal communication.

Research on the speech and language of individuals with MR has been carried out using subjects in special schools, institutions, clinics, and other service settings. In a recent review by Dodd and Lechy (1989), estimates of speech impediments in populations with MR ranged from 25 percent to 95 percent, depending on the criteria used and the population tested. The authors further state that "a variety of factors determine the degree of severity and type of . . . disorder . . . [mainly] . . . cause of handicap, degree of cognitive impairment and type of care" (p. 36). Mittler (1974) suggests that language difficulties in people with MR indicate "underfunctioning in relation to their level of skills in other areas of development" (p. 527). Thus, the problems with language in populations with MR may be greater than one might expect. No attention has been paid to verbal communication in epidemiological studies of representative populations of people with MR, except for a study carried out by Gould (1976) in the former London borough of Camberwell. On the census day (December 31, 1970), all children in Camberwell up to age 14 who had severe MR (IQ <50) were identified (*n* 150). Those with no language were differentiated from those with some language. For the age groups 0–4, 5–9, and 10–14 years, 51 percent, 37 percent, and 43 percent, respectively, had no language . Gould presented a careful discussion of factors related to lack of language development and concluded that an organic explanation was more likely than an environmental one.

The Follow-up Study

Our purpose in developing the measures for the present study was to obtain relatively simple, straightforward estimates of young people's abilities in verbal communication. We made no attempt to use the many technical forms of assessment that have been developed in the field of speech and language research. The measure of verbal communication we developed had two components, language usage and speech impediments, based on the speech and language used by respondents during their interview, (which had a median length of approximately three hours). As part of their overall intensive training, interviewers noted their observations on informants' language usage and speech impediments, and their interview performance was monitored and evaluated (see Chapter 4). Although the use of a single interviewer for each interview session precluded reliability tests of the ratings, it is reasonable to expect, as a result of the training and monitoring of the interviewers and because the ratings were simple and required no technical skills, that at least a fair degree of validity was obtained.

Our analysis is based on interviews with 170 young people, who comprised 81 percent of the 211 survivors.

1. *Language Usage.* Language usage was based on the informant's vocabulary, comprehension of questions, and quality of responses, according to the following scales:

Vocabulary: (1) Very good and Good; (2) Average; (3) Fair; (4) Very limited; (5) Striking absence of words.

Comprehension: (1) Very good and Good; (2) Average; (3) Fair; (4) Very limited.

Quality of response: (1) Full; (2) Adequate; (3) Limited; (4) Severely limited.

If it was not possible to elicit any information relevant to the interviewer's questions, or if the person being interviewed had no speech, or virtually no speech, the interviewer described the ways in which the person did or did not communicate verbally.

For the study subjects with MR, the correlations among the three ratings—vocabulary, comprehension, and quality of response—ranged from 0.64 to 0.76. Because the correlations were high, the ratings were summed, giving a range of scores of language usage of 3 to 13. For ease of analysis, these scores were then converted to a range of 1 to 11, with 1 representing the best language usage and 11 the poorest. A score of 12 was assigned to subjects having no or virtually no speech.

Using the scale of 1 to 11, we developed three categories of language usage for further use in measuring verbal communication. To do this, we examined language usage among the nonretarded comparisons and found that 93 percent had scores of 3 or less. Most of the young adults with a score of 3 had average vocabulary, good comprehension, and adequate quality of response. We then combined the three components and assigned the following categories: 1–3, Good; 4–5, Fair; and 6–11, Poor.

2. *Speech Impediments.* The purpose of this rating was to assess the extent to which speech impediments were obstacles in verbal intercourse. We made no attempt to rate specific impediments. For individuals with no language, clearly, speech impediments could not be evaluated. For those with some language, interviewers circled either "yes" or "no" for each of the following: Speech unclear? Speech slurred? Lisp? Speech impediment? Other problem with speech? For each "yes" response, the interviewer then wrote a full description, and these were evaluated by two judges, who considered the extent to which verbal communication was impeded, distorted, or made unclear, or the extent to which it was difficult to understand the informant. Disagreements between judges were resolved through discussion or the opinion of a third judge. In their descriptions, interviewers used terms such as *lisp, stammer, stutter, rapid,* and *indistinct.* The judges rated the evidence for speech impediments as follows:

None: no evidence of any speech impediment.

Mild: only a single impediment was noted, described as slight or mild, or occurring only occasionally.

Moderate: an impediment was described without qualification; or more than one kind of impediment was described, and these were qualified as slight, mild, or occasional: or the combination of descriptive terms indicated an overall moderate degree of impediment to understanding.

Severe: an impediment was described using adjectives such as severe, bad, or poor; or multiple impediments were described that together seriously hindered understanding the informant.

3. *Verbal Communication.* To obtain an overall measure of verbal communication, we combined the ratings on language usage and speech impediments. Individuals who had no speech, or virtually no speech, were kept in a separate category. If some speech was present, we assigned a rating of *poor verbal communication disorder* if both poor use of language and a moderate or severe speech impediment were present, and a rating of *moderate* if only one of these was present (that is, either language usage was poor or there was a moderate to severe speech impediment). Individuals with fair language usage and mild speech impediments, alone or together, were not rated as having a disorder of verbal communication.

We found the following:

1. *Language Usage.* The association between IQ and language usage is well known, in part, because the assessment of language skills is an aspect of intelligence tests. It was thus expected that among the young adults with MR, the higher the IQ, the better the language usage. Although in the follow-up study, the IQ's were obtained in childhood and the assessment of language usage was made when the subjects were aged 22, our expectation of a high correlation between IQ in childhood and language usage at age 22 was confirmed (Pearson $r = -.76$). When the analysis was limited to those in the population with mild MR (IQ 50+), the correlation dropped to $-.45$ but remained significant. This drop reflects the very high correlation for those with severe MR.

Throughout the study, we were interested in whether the personal characteristics of those members of the study population with IQ's of 70 and above, who might not have been classified as MR under current definitions, were different from those with IQ's of 60 to 69. A one-way Analysis of Variance (ANOVA) to examine differences in language usage among the four IQ groups (IQ <50, 50–59, 60–69, and 70+) was highly significant ($F = 64.49$, $p = .000$). The analysis combined males and females because no gender differences were found. Table 10.1 shows the means and standard deviations on which the ANOVA was based. Language usage improved as IQ increased up to IQ 60–69. A post hoc Least Significant Difference procedure showed that the three IQ groups of <50, 50–59, and 60–69 were all significantly different from one another, but that there was no significant difference between those with IQ 60–69 and 70+.

All those with no speech had an IQ below 50, and significantly more were male than female (Table 10.2). Of the ten males with no speech, seven had spent most of their lives in institutional care, with age at entry ranging from 2 to 9 years. Two had Down syndrome, seven had cerebral palsy, and one had a severe hearing loss.

2. *Speech Impediments.* Our examination of speech impediments was restricted to those who had some speech (1–11 on the scale of language usage). Since no gender differences were found, we combined males and females. Of the 157 young adults with some speech, impediments were mild for 16 percent, moderate for 19 percent, and severe for 8 percent (see Table 10.3). Most (57 percent) had no

Table 10.1 Means and standard deviation (SD) on the scale of language usage for the population with mental retardation by IQ group

IQ	*N*	Mean[a]	SD
<50	38	9.29	2.71
50–59	35	5.60	2.26
60–69	59	4.03	1.65
70+	37	3.62	1.50

a. A score of 1 indicated the best language usage and a score of 11, the poorest, with a score of 12 indicating no speech.

Table 10.2 Presence and absence of speech in males and females with IQ's below 50

Subjects with IQ's below 50	Speech present	Speech absent
Males	11	10
Females	14	2

$\chi^2 = 6.11$, $df = 1$, $p < .025$.

Table 10.3 Speech impediments by IQ group for the population with mental retardation

	Level of impediment							
	None		Mild		Moderate		Severe	
IQ	*N*	(%)	*N*	(%)	*N*	(%)	*N*	(%)
<50	8	(32)	4	(16)	3	(12)	10	(40)
50–59	15	(40)	7	(20)	13	(37)	0	
60–69	41	(70)	10	(17)	8	(14)	0	
70+	26	(68)	4	(11)	6	(16)	2	(5)
Total	90	(57)	25	(16)	30	(19)	12	(8)

$\chi^2 = 55.10$, df $= 9$, $p = .0000$.

speech impediments, which decreased as IQ increased across the three groups from IQ <50 to 60–69. As we found for language usage, there was no difference between those with IQ 60–69 and 70+. In fact, the only severe speech impediments among those with IQ 50+ were found in two young adults with IQ's over 70.

3. *Verbal Communication (this measure combined language usage and speech impediments).* The greater difficulties with verbal communication among people with MR compared to nonretarded peers is well known. What is not known is how many people with MR have abilities in verbal communication that are within the range of nonretarded peers. This question is of greatest relevance to those young adults who disappeared from MR services after leaving school. These are the young people about whom least is known, because they are most likely to be missed in studies of adults with MR seen in clinical or service facilities. In the present study, the young adults who disappeared from services comprise 72 percent of all those with mild MR.

Table 10.4 shows the verbal communication for all the young adults with MR by IQ group, for the subgroup with mild MR (IQ 50+) who disappeared from services, and for the nonretarded comparison population. Males and females were combined because we found no gender differences aside from that already shown between males and females with severe MR (IQ <50). As in the separate ratings of language usage and speech impediments, there were statistically significant differences in verbal communication between each of the contiguous IQ groups except IQ 60–69 and 70+. What is of greater

Table 10.4 Verbal communication in the study population

Verbal communication disorder	Young adults with mental retardation								IQ 50+, no services		Comparisons	
	IQ <50		50–59		60–69		70+					
	N = 38	(%)	N = 35	(%)	N = 59	(%)	N = 37	(%)	N = 94	(%)	N = 149	(%)
None	0		10	(29)	42	(71)	28	(76)	66	(70)	139	(93)
Moderate	14	(37)	18	(51)	17	(29)	7	(19)	24	(26)	10	(7)
Severe	12	(32)	7	(20)	0		2	(5)	4	(4)	0	
No speech	12	(32)	0		0		0		0		0	

IQ <50 vs. 50–59: $\chi^2 = 22.92$, df = 3, $p < .001$.
IQ 50–59 vs. 60–69: $\chi^2 = 25.51$, df = 2, $p < .001$.
IQ 60–69 vs. 70+: $\chi^2 = 3.88$, df = 2, n.s.
IQ 50+, no services vs. comparisons: $\chi^2 = 24.57$, df = 2, $p < .001$.

interest is that the young adults who disappeared from services had significantly more problems in verbal communication than the comparisons, although 70 percent of the former had no verbal communication disorder.

The results show the extent of the problems that young people with MR have in verbal communication. Skill in verbal communication is basic for social interactions, both during and outside working hours. The next chapter considers verbal communication in the context of other disabilities.

11

Patterns of Disability

Mental retardation (MR) has been defined as an impairment of intelligence that results in disabilities in areas such as knowledge acquisition, education, personal safety, and situational behavior (World Health Organization [WHO], 1980). MR may, in addition, be the result of an impairment of the central nervous system that is also a cause of other disabling conditions, such as cerebral palsy and epilepsy. In a manual of classification, the WHO attempted to clarify the terms *impairment, disability,* and *handicap,* using the following definitions:

> *Impairment* is any loss or abnormality of psychological, physiological, or anatomical structure or function . . .
> *Disability* is any restriction or lack (resulting from an impairment) of ability to perform an activity in the manner or within the range considered normal for a human being . . .
> *Handicap* is a disadvantage for a given individual, resulting from an impairment or a disability, that limits or prevents the fulfillment of a role that is normal (depending on age, sex, and social and cultural factors) for that individual. (pp. 27–29)

This chapter will deal only with disabilities. We will summarize the frequencies found for each disability, consider the patterns of disability as they occurred among the young adults with MR, and examine the total degree of disability experienced by each person. The analyses build on a previously published report (Richardson et al., 1984b).

In earlier chapters, we reported higher rates of behavior disturbance and verbal communication disorders among the young people with MR than among the nonretarded comparison population, and we reported a higher rate of epilepsy than has been found in general populations. Other studies have shown a strong relationship between cerebral palsy (CP) and MR (Susser et al., 1985). In Chapter 6, on etiology, we used CP as a marker of underlying brain injury that was the presumed common cause of both the MR and the CP.

Few epidemiologic studies, however, provide information on how disabilities combine in individuals with MR. One important study, carried out by Rutter, Tizard, and Whitmore (1970), showed how physical and psychiatric handicap combined in children with intellectual and educational handicap on the Isle of Wight. Their definition of intellectual handicap was a psychometric definition of MR. They found that "one third of the intellectually retarded had a physical handicap (most often . . . a neurological condition which was probably the primary cause of their retardation) and more than a fifth had a psychiatric disability." They concluded that, "As only one in ten of the intellectually retarded had no other handicap, it is abundantly clear that most intellectually handicapped children present multiple problems" (p. 353). Comparisons between their study, which considered children, and our analysis of young adults must be made with caution.

In the Wessex survey of children and adults with MR (reported in Kushlick and Blunden 1974), Kushlick and his associates looked at three conditions that required special care: behavior disturbance, nonambulation, and incontinence. Only behavior disturbance can be related to our study. Their survey was based on health register data, which included virtually all individuals with severe MR but only a small proportion of those with mild MR. Kushlick and Blunden reported that "by age 15 to 19, 71 per cent of severely subnormal people are continent, ambulant, and with no severe behavior disorders." "This," they suggested, "is because some of the children with the most severe incapacities die, while others make progress" (p. 45).

In a recent epidemiologic study of 10-year-old children in Atlanta, Georgia, Murphy et al. (1995) examined four disabilities coexisting with MR—CP, epilepsy, and impaired vision and hearing. Among the children with mild MR, 12 percent had one or more of these disabilities—6 percent had CP, 7 percent had epilepsy, and 2 percent had sensory impairments. Among the children with severe MR, 45 percent had one or more disabilities—28 percent had CP, 32 percent had epilepsy, and 11 percent had sensory impairments. These researchers did not examine behavior disturbance, and they dealt only with children, but the prevalence rates for severe and mild MR were similar to those in the our study, making comparison useful.

The Follow-up Study

The degree of central nervous system impairment that results in severe MR often results in other disabling conditions as well, while individuals with mild MR less often have these accompanying disabilities. Therefore, we will examine these two groups separately. The analysis is for the postschool years, ages 16 to 22, because the data were most complete for that period. We had complete data on disabilities for 171 study subjects, 95 males and 76 females.

The analysis was limited to moderately-to-severely disabling impairments: motor disabilities and those due to epilepsy, behavior disturbance, vision and hearing losses, and verbal communication disorders. We obtained information on physical disabilities and behavior disturbance from medical and social work records, and from interviews and observations of study subjects and their parents.

Motor disabilities were due mainly to CP, and ratings were based on the degree of functional limitations. Disability due to epilepsy was based on the frequency of seizures and the severity of symptoms (see Chapter 8 for a description of behavior disturbance ratings and Chapter 9 for epilepsy definitions). Total deafness was rated as severe, and hearing losses that caused problems in communication as moderate. Impairments of vision included were total blindness, rated as a severe disability, and lack of sight in one eye, rated as moderate. No other visual impairments found in the population caused much disability. For verbal communication disorders (see Chapter 10), lack of any real speech was considered a severe disability. If the person had both poor use of language and a moderate or severe speech impediment, the resulting verbal communication disorder was also rated as a severe disability. If language usage was poor or there was a moderate or severe speech impediment, a rating of moderate was given.

We found the following:

The frequency and severity of each disability, in addition to MR, are shown in Table 11.1. With the exception of behavior disturbance, all occurred less often among those with mild MR than with severe MR.

Among those with severe MR, verbal communication disorders were present for everyone, behavior disturbance and motor disabilities each affected about a third, epilepsy occurred somewhat less often, and disabilities due to vision and hearing loss were infrequent. Among those with mild MR, behavior disturbance (moderate and severe combined) and moderate verbal communication disorders were most frequent.

The types of disabilities for each individual as they occurred, singly and in combination, are shown in Table 11.2 (in order to make the data manageable, we combined moderate and severe disabilities). Among young adults with severe MR, a verbal communications disorder was the only disability that occurred alone, and it was found

Table 11.1 Percentages of moderate and severe disabilities for young adults with severe (IQ <50) and mild (IQ 50+) mental retardation

Disability	IQ <50 (N = 37)	IQ 50+ (N = 134)
VC disorder[a]		
Moderate	35	34
Severe	65	7
Behavior disturbance		
Moderate	14	14
Severe	16	23
Motor disabilities		
Moderate	19	6
Severe	14	2
Epilepsy		
Moderate	11	5
Severe	11	2
Vision		
Moderate	5	0
Severe	3	0
Hearing		
Moderate	3	1
Severe	3	0

a. VC–Verbal communications.

Table 11.2 Percentages with various combinations of moderate and severe disabilities for young adults with severe (IQ <50) and mild (IQ 50+) mental retardation

	IQ <50		IQ 50+	
	(*N* = 37)	(%)	(*N* = 134)	(%)
No Moderate or Severe Disability	0		46	(34)
Single Disability				
Motor (M)	0		2	(1.5)
Epilepsy (E)	0		2	(1.5)
Behavior disturbance (BD)	0		28	(22)
Verbal comm. disorder (VC)	13	(35)	25	(19)
Hearing (H)	0		1	(1)
Vision (V)	0		0	
Total	13	(35)	58	(43)
Two Disabilities				
M and E	0		1	(<1)
M and BD	0		1	(<1)
M and VC	4	(11)	2	(1.5)
E and BD	0		1	(<1)
E and VC	3	(8)	1	(<1)
BD and VC	6	(16)	16	(12)
VC and V	1	(<3)	0	
VC and H	1	(<3)	1	(<1)
Total	15	(41)	23	(17)
Three or More Disabilities				
M and E and VC	3	(8)	3	(2)
M and BD and VC	3	(8)	2	(1.5)
M and VC and H	1	(<3)	0	
E and BD and VC	1	(<3)	2	(1.5)
M and E and VC and V	1	(<3)	0	
Total	9	(24)	7	(5)

for more than a third. The most frequent combinations were verbal communication disorders combined with behavior disturbance (16 percent) and with motor disabilities (11 percent). A quarter of those with severe MR had three or more additional disabilities.

By contrast, among the young adults with mild MR, a third had no moderate or severe disability, nearly a half had a single disability, and less than a quarter had multiple disabilities. As might be expected from Table 11.1, behavior disturbance and verbal communication disorders, both alone and in combination, stand out as the most common disabilities.

Other Disabilities

Two other disabling conditions, not considered in the analysis, affected some members of the study population. Two young adults with mild MR had heart conditions whose symptoms were disabling, and both also had other moderate disabilities. Daytime incontinence occurred in three young adults with severe MR and three with mild MR. Five of the six were severely disabled by other conditions, while one had no other disabilities.

Down Syndrome

Down syndrome is one of the most common and easily recognizable biomedical diagnoses found in populations with MR, and disabilities among people with Down syndrome may be of special interest. Eight individuals survived to age 22. One, with mild MR, had a moderate verbal communication disorder. The remaining seven, with severe MR, all had a severe verbal communications disorder, one was also blind in one eye, and another had severe behavior disturbance.

Disabilities among Subjects with Missing Data

Among study subjects with severe MR, data were missing for nine. Only three survived past childhood. By the time of the follow-up, all had died, and their parents were not interviewed. Since all study subjects with severe MR for whom we had complete data had a verbal communication disorder, it is likely that those who died did also. We do not know whether any of them had behavior disturbance, but one was known to have had epilepsy, two had CP, and three had Down syndrome.

Among study subjects with mild MR, data were missing for forty-one. Two had committed suicide at age 18, and the remainder refused to participate in the study or were not traced. No verbal communications data and only partial behavior disturbance data were available for these young people.

There was nothing here to suggest that missing data biased the results, and we felt confident that the data presented in Tables 11.1 and 11.2 were fairly representative of the whole study population.

The patterns of disabilities shown in Table 11.2 give some indication of the total extent to which individuals in the study could be considered disabled, but moderate and severe disabilities are combined. A somewhat better indication of the severity of disabling conditions is shown in Table 11.3, although the type of disability is not shown. We placed the degree of disability in a general hierarchy according to multiplicity and severity—from no disabilities to multiple severe disabilities—but we made no assumption of an exact ordering of the degree of overall disability at adjacent levels within the table. Single severe disabilities appear in the table below multiple moderate disabilities, for example, but people in the first group may not be more disabled than people in the second.

As one would expect from the previous tables, the degree of disability was far greater among those with severe MR than those with mild MR. Single severe disabilities affected similar proportions of the young adults with severe and mild MR, but there were major differences in type of disability. For the young adults with severe MR, the single disability was always in verbal communication, whereas for almost all those with mild MR it was due to behavior disturbance.

The following examples of how the addition of disabilities to MR impinged on the lives of the young adults and their families are useful in showing how the data presented relate to individuals.

Sharon had mild MR. Her speech was not clear, and her words

Table 11.3 Multiplicity and severity of disabilities (in percent) for young adults with severe (IQ <50) and mild (IQ 50+) mental retardation

Disabilities	IQ <50 (*N* = 37)	IQ 50+ (*N* = 134)
1. No disability (or mild only)	0	34
2. Single moderate disability	13	28
3. Multiple moderate disabilities	19	8
4. Single severe disability	22	16
5. Single severe and one of the more moderate disabilities	19	10
6. Multiple severe disabilities	27	4

often slurred together. In addition, she was often inattentive and uninterested in the interviewer's questions, and these two factors made interviewing her difficult. She was obsessively concerned with an imaginary rash on her hand and with dryness and a bad taste in her mouth (side effects of medication). At age 22, Sharon was hospitalized for depression. She had become extremely upset and refused to go to the adult day care center she had attended for several years. Her disturbed emotional state and her language difficulties caused problems for her and her family beyond those due to her mental retardation.

Raymond could walk short distances with assistance, but he spent most of the day in a wheelchair. His left hand was immobilized in a bent position, he had a hearing loss, and he could not communicate with speech. When his sister came to visit him in the institution where he lived, however, his smile and gestures demonstrated his delight at seeing her. Raymond's mental retardation was severe, but his other disabilities had been important factors leading to his institutionalization.

Donald was immobile: if placed on the ground in a seated position he could remain that way, but he could not pull himself up into a seated position if he was lying down and had to be lifted in and out of his wheelchair. He had no speech at all, and did not acknowledge the presence of the interviewer in any way. As severe as these disabilities were, epilepsy caused even greater problems. He had been on several different medications, but none controlled the seizures. At times, he would have several seizures in one day, and at other times, he would go a few days without any. He slept in his parents' bedroom, so that they could give him immediate attention if he had a seizure during the night. Donald's parents devoted their lives to his care, but it took a heavy toll on their mental and physical health.

Summary and Comparisons with Other Studies

Verbal communication disorders were found among all those in the study population with severe MR and among 41 percent of those with mild MR. Despite these high rates, and the importance of verbal communication in everyday living, few studies have noted its frequency, and the three epidemiologic studies noted earlier took no account of them. What we found in the follow-up study was that when two or more additional disabilities were present together, the most frequent combination was behavior disturbance and verbal communication disorders. Among the young adults with mild MR, behavior disturbance was the most common disability.

To the extent that comparison of our data with those presented by Rutter, Tizard, and Whitmore (1970) are meaningful, we found lower rates of physical disability and higher rates of behavior disturbance. About a third of the children with intellectual retardation in the Isle of Wight study had a physical disability, which the authors defined as chronic physical disorders (lasting a year or more) associated with some kind of persistent or recurrent handicap that was present at the time of the survey. They included disorders such as asthma, epilepsy, cerebral palsy, diabetes, and heart disease. Because their definition was broader than ours, it is not surprising that the young adults in our follow-up study had fewer physical disabilities than the children in the Isle of Wight study, even if we include all but verbal communication disorders and behavior disturbance. In addition, we did not take mild disabilities into account. Rutter, Tizard, and Whitmore reported that more than a fifth of the children with intellectual retardation also had a psychiatric disorder. In our follow-up study, more than a third of the young adults had moderate-to-severe behavior disturbance. Some of this difference is probably because Rutter and colleagues limited their evaluations to a short period prior to the study, whereas our behavior disturbance ratings took account of the entire seven-year postschool period.

Kushlick and Blunden (1974) reported that 29 percent of the adults with severe MR in their Wessex study were incontinent, nonambulant, or had behavior disturbance. It seems reasonable that the percentage with behavior disturbance would be lower than that, since some of that 29 percent were incontinent or nonambulant but did not have behavior disturbance. In our study, 30 percent of the young people with severe MR had behavior disturbance (see Table 11.1), which is higher than the probable percentage in the Wessex study. In addition, if verbal communication disorders are discounted, 65 percent of the young adults with severe MR in our study had at least one other moderate or severe disability (see Table 11.2), more than double the rate of disability in the Wessex study. That study did not include ambulatory motor disabilities or epilepsy, however, which were included in our follow-up.

Because Murphy et al. (1995) did not include behavior disturbance or verbal communication disorders among the associated disabilities they examined in their Atlanta study, the proportions of children in that study with disabilities were much lower than ours. But when we compared specific types of disability, the proportions were similar, although the Atlanta study looked at children and ours at adults, and we noted only moderate and severe disabilities. Among those with mild MR, Murphy et al. found that 6 percent had CP, 7 percent had epilepsy, and 2 percent had sensory impairments (vision and hearing). Our findings were almost identical (see Table 11.1). Among those with severe MR, the Atlanta study found 28 percent with CP, 32 percent with epilepsy, and 11 percent with sensory impairments. Except for epilepsy,the results were again very similar. The lower rate of epilepsy among the young people with severe MR in the follow-up study was due to our exclusion of those with only mild disability due to the epilepsy. When we examined the rate of all epilepsy among those with severe MR (see Chapter 6 on etiology), it was 35 percent, in line with the Atlanta study.

To understand the lives of young people with MR, it is clear that the additional disabilities with which they and their parents or caretakers need to cope must be taken into account.

12

Appearance

A persistent theme in literature and drama, now supported by a growing body of research, is that people's appearance influences both their self-concept and their relationships with others (see Richardson, Koller, and Katz 1985c for a more comprehensive report). *Beauty and the Beast, The Hunchback of Notre Dame, The Elephant Man,* and *Cyrano de Bergerac* all portray characters whose unattractive exterior masks sensitivity and intelligence.

To explain how people respond to atypical appearance, Richardson (1976) suggested that atypical characteristics violate normative expectations of how people should appear. During socialization, we develop an increasingly complex set of normative expectations, or schema, about how people should appear in their dress, manner, speech, movement, and behavior. We become accustomed to some variability, but when we encounter someone whose appearance, manner, or behavior exceeds the limits of our expectations, we react with emotional arousal, anxiety, and fear, and behave differently toward that person. The evidence supporting the concept of violation of expectation and the nature of these changes in behavior (Richardson 1968, 1976, 1983; Wright 1983) as well as research that focuses on physical attractiveness and unattractiveness are reviewed elsewhere (Adams 1977; Berscheid and Walster 1974; Bull and Rumsey 1988). What the research suggests, in brief, is that an atypical appearance creates a social obstacle that places a person at a disadvantage, especially in the initial phases of social encounters.

Physical appearance is made up of many components, including body size, structure, proportions, facial configuration, movement, hair, dress, grooming, posture, gestures, and mannerisms. Most investigators dealing with physical appearance have varied a single component while holding constant or randomizing others. No investigators have examined various combinations of attractiveness and atypicality or combined several components of appearance into a summary measure.

There are several reasons for expecting a more atypical appearance among people with mental retardation (MR) than among nonretarded individuals, and for expecting that atypical appearance increases with increasing severity of mental retardation. Central nervous system (CNS) impairment can cause atypical movement, posture, facial expressions, and gestures. Virtually all individuals with severe MR, but only about 25 percent of those with mild MR, have CNS impairment (Birch et al. 1970; Tarjan 1970). Factors that lead to prenatal CNS impairment may also influence cranial and facial growth (Israel 1980). Specific genetic disorders sometimes cause identifying facial signs, as in Down syndrome, epiloia, Apert syndrome, cretinism, and Crouzon disease (Berg 1974).

Behavior disturbance, seizures, and disorders of movement, speech, hearing, and vision tend to increase in both degree and frequency with severity of MR (see Chapters 8, 9, and 10). Side effects of treatment with anticonvulsant and psychotropic drugs may also contribute to atypical appearance, as may muscle contractures and the repetitive stereotypical behavior found among some people with severe MR (Berkson 1983).

Experiential and social factors may also cause individuals with MR to appear atypical. In families where intellectual impairment is prevalent, for example, there may be atypical customs, habits, or behavior that are reflected in appearance. Tarjan (1970) suggested that children with MR attributable to sociocultural factors who disappear from mental retardation services as adults are normal in appearance, but there is no research evidence to support this suggestion. Mutual imitation in an institution may lead to conspicuous atypicality after transfer to a community residence (Birenbaum and Seiffer 1976), even though some of these forms of behavior may have been appropriate and even adaptive in the institutional setting. Atypical appearance can be a barrier to social intercourse, causing isolation and maladaptive behavior that may tip judgment toward classifying a borderline child as MR.

In this chapter we describe methods used to rate atypical appearance, consider the distribution of the measure in the study population by testing various hypotheses that relate appearance to CNS impairment, and examine whether young adults with mild MR who disappeared from mental retardation services differ in appearance from nonretarded peers.

Measures

Indicators of Central Nervous System (CNS) Impairment

The degree of mental retardation, using IQ, was employed as one indicator of CNS impairment. Virtually all individuals with IQ's below 50 have some CNS impairment (Birch et al. 1970). Some have genetic and biochemical abnormalities that have specific physical stigmata, such as Down syndrome. Among those with IQ's 50 and above, the proportion with CNS impairment decreases as IQ increases (Koller, Richardson, and Katz 1984).

A second indicator was actual CNS status. This was identified using the neurological examination obtained in the earlier study (Birch et al. 1970; see Chapter 1) for the children born in 1952 to 1954 who received MR services in 1962.

History of Adult Mental Retardation Services

A history of adult mental retardation services was obtained for all study subjects (see Richardson et al. 1984a; see also Chapter 15). On the basis of this information, we subdivided the young adults with mild MR into two groups: those who received MR services for more than two-thirds of the period from age 16 to 22 (n = 38) and those who received either no MR services or minimal services (n = 80). This measure was used to examine the question of whether young adults with MR who received services had a more atypical appearance than those who did not.

Appearance

The selection of components of atypical appearance was influenced by several considerations: the components should be relatively enduring; they should include the range of cues expected to be important in interpersonal evaluation, including dynamic as well as static features; and they should be restricted to those likely to be barriers to interpersonal relations. It was clear that photographs would be inadequate, because they are static and provide only a momentary glimpse of an individual's appearance. We obtained appearance data instead from the interviewers' observations (see Chapter 4). Certainly, their observations were not independent of their knowledge of the informants, but neither are observations made in everyday life situations. Interviewers did not know the IQ's of informants.

After the interview, the interviewers reviewed lists of atypicalities in the observation schedule, checked off any that were present, and wrote descriptions for those checked. The checklist included *facial characteristics* (tics, twitches, paralysis, grimaces, asymmetry, drooling, unusual features, other), *other bodily features* (physical handicaps, proportions, use of prosthesis, posture, bitten nails, other), and *movement* (spasticity, clumsiness, gait, mannerisms, gestures, other). Interviewers also circled one for each of the following scales: *facial appearance:* good looking, average, ugly (the word *ugly* was used to remind interviewers only to use the rating for those with extremely unattractive faces); *weight for height:* obese, overweight, average, underweight, very thin; *Height:* very tall (males over 6'2"; females over 5'11"), tall (males, 5'10"–6'2"; females, 5'7"–5'10"), average (males, 5'6"–5'9"; females, 5'3"–5'7"), small (males, 5'0"–5'5"; females, 4'11"–5'2"), very small (males, less than 5'0"; females, less than 4'11").

Components of Atypical Appearance

From interviewers' written descriptions we made a set of components of atypical appearance that was influenced by the literature we reviewed. Each component was rated on a scale of 0 to 3 (absent, slight, moderate, severe). Following are the definitions of each component and the instructions given to coders, as well as several examples and how they were rated:

Atypical facial characteristics. Evidence may derive from eyes, nose, ears, chin, mouth, teeth, tongue, forehead, facial hair (female), asymmetry, and baldness, but not hair style. Tics and twitches should be coded under movement, and a large or small head under proportions. Examples of descriptions and their ratings: *Slight*—(a) a soft, round, chubby face, rather effeminate; (b) very deep-set eyes. *Mod-*

erate—(a) lower lip and jaw protruded; (b) eyes different in size and shape. *Severe*—(a) eyes constantly moved, no teeth, head misshapen; (b) eyes close together, forehead sloped back, head pointed.

Atypical expressions and manner. These convey or are commonly interpreted as signifying some inappropriate feeling, state, emotion, or mood, whether or not deliberately intended. Examples of descriptions and their ratings: *Slight*—(a) rather awkward and still, but I think through shyness; (b) screwed up his face sometimes before he answered. *Moderate*—(a) picked his nose quite unconsciously; (b) picked his skin around nails until one of them bled. *Severe*—(a) stared into space, oblivious of interviewer sometimes, sucked lower lip, rocked backwards and forward a lot, and waved arms throughout interview; (b) made faces, eyes half- closed when relaxed, pointed when required something, banged arm of chair to attract attention.

Atypical expressions and deformities. These are deviations from normal body proportions or presence of some bodily deformity. Obesity is not included here, as it was coded separately. Examples: *Slight*—Small feet. *Moderate*—Slight hunchback; unusually long arms and fingers. *Severe*—A massive head compared with rest of body.

Atypical movement. Atypical movements should largely be outside the control of the person and include facial twitches, tics, and tremors. Examples of descriptions and their ratings: *Slight*—(a) Slight tremor in hands; (b) rather slow. *Moderate*—(a) movement very slow and shuffled; (b) all movements slow and deliberate. *Severe*—(a) left arm and leg paralyzed, limped when walking due to paralyzed leg; (b) can hardly use hand at all, drags one leg a little as he walks, couldn't sit still and made continuous jerky movements all the time.

Skin conditions. A single boil or a few pimples are probably temporary and should not be included. Severe acne is likely to be chronic. Skin color that deviates from the norms of the community should be included. Examples: *Slight*—Acne on face. *Moderate*—Poor skin, many spots, boils developing on lower jaw. *Severe*—(a) skin very bad, boils, acne; (b) large birthmark covers over half of face.

Scars. Scars are judged by their prominence and location and any reference to size and severity. Examples: *Slight*—scarred hand. *Moderate*—scarred left cheek. *Severe*—neck was noticeably and extensively scarred on the right side up to her chin, and the left side of the neck was slightly scarred.

Age-appearance discrepancy. This relates to appearance that deviates from what is expected for chronological age (22 years). Ratings are based on the amount of emphasis given by the observer, and only slight and moderate are used. For example: *Slight*—looked somewhat younger than 22. *Moderate*—looked about 35 to 40 years old.

Drooling. Any reference to drooling is rated moderate or severe. For example: *Moderate*—drools slightly when talking excitedly. *Severe*—drools fairly constantly.

Severely bitten nails and *Glasses with thick lenses* are rated as slight; *Appearance of Down syndrome* is rated as moderate.

Other. The characteristics of ugly, obese, or very small (males) are rated as severe; very small for females is rated as slight.

Coding of Components

Each observation schedule was coded independently by two people. Subjects' IQ's were not known to the coders. Disagreements were resolved between the coders, but if a difference remained, a third person coded the data independently, and a final decision was arrived at by consensus. For the components that required judgment, Kappa values (Fleiss, Cohen, and Everitt 1969) were used to measure reliability between the first two independent codings. Four of the Kappa values obtained ranged from 0.88 to 1.0, indicating excellent agreement. An additional four ranged from 0.54 to 0.67, indicating fair to good agreement. Reliability on coding of atypical facial characteristics had an unsatisfactory Kappa level of 0.48. We retained this component in the study because of the consensus system used in arriving at all final judgments.

The two components that dealt with the face, atypical facial characteristics and ugly facial appearance, were kept separate on conceptual grounds. It was possible, however, that the measures heavily overlapped, introducing unnecessary redundance. On examining the relationship between the two components for the total population with MR, we found that, of the 72 percent with no atypicalities of the face, 16 percent were rated as ugly; of the 28 percent who had an atypical face, 23 percent were rated as ugly. It seemed justified, then, to keep the two components because they were sufficiently separate. There was, however, an increase in ratings of ugly as ratings of facial atypicality became more severe.

Summary measure. After the components had been coded separately, the scores were summed for each subject to give a summary atypical appearance measure. To determine the appropriateness of summing the components, we estimated the internal consistency to be 0.65 using Cronbach's alpha coefficient, indicating moderate to good internal consistency. No significant change occurred in the alpha coefficient when any one of the components was deleted, indicating the stability of Cronbach's alpha coefficient with the given components.

The following hypotheses were tested to explore the relationship between the summary measure of atypical appearance and the indicators of CNS impairment.

Hypothesis 1: Atypical appearance will increase with severity of MR. Table 12.1 shows the means, standard deviations, and ranges of summary atypical appearance scores for young adults grouped by degree of mental retardation. An analysis of variance, with the summary atypical appearance measure as the dependent variable, showed a significant main effect, $F(3,166) = 23.18$, $p = .0000$. The Least Significant Difference procedure then showed significant differences between each adjacent IQ group except between IQ 60–69 and 70+. The results support the hypothesis that atypical appearance increases with severity of mental retardation.

Hypothesis 2: Among people with mild MR, those with evidence of CNS impairment will be more atypical in appearance than those without. The hypothesis was tested on subjects with mild MR (IQ 50+) using the results of the neurological examination given to three birth cohorts of 1952–1954, when they were aged 8 to 10 years. We found that those with evidence of CNS impairment were significantly more atypical in appearance than those without such evidence ($t[48] = 3.11$, $p < .005$).

Table 12.1 Mean, standard deviation (SD), and range of atypical appearance summary scores by IQ group

IQ	*N*	Mean[a]	SD	Range
<50	37	5.84	3.62	0–16
50–59	36	3.53	3.24	0–12
60–69	60	1.72	1.87	0–8
70+	37	1.62	1.62	0–6

a. Low scores indicate less atypical appearance and high scores indicate more.

Hypothesis 3: People with mild MR who receive adult mental retardation services will be more atypical in appearance than those who manage without such services. This hypothesis has both biological and social bases. First, adults with mild MR who receive services often do so because of associated disabilities rather than on grounds of intellectual disability alone. Second, adults in services spend a major part of their time with other people with MR and may imitate certain behavior that leads to atypical appearance. We found those with IQ's 50 and above in adult services were significantly more atypical in appearance than those in the same IQ range who had not been in adult mental retardation services ($t[116] = 4.9, p < 001$).

Confirmation of these three hypotheses gave us confidence that the summary measure of atypical appearance had some veracity. The final step toward this end was to examine whether this measure of appearance was indeed atypical; that is, whether it occurred rarely among the young nonretarded adults chosen as comparisons (see Chapter 4). We felt this was an important step, because the measure was not empirically derived from a survey of the general population but from a conceptualization based on related research literature. We therefore examined the distribution of the summary atypical appearance measure in the nonretarded comparison population and found that 70 percent had no indicators of atypical appearance (that is, had a score of 0), 19 percent had a score of 1, and 11 percent had a score of 2 or 3.

We felt the measure could now be used to determine whether there were differences in appearance between the young adults with mild MR who received no adult mental retardation services and matched comparisons. No clear evidence was available from previous research or theory on which to base a hypothesis, although Tarjan (1970) suggested that there would be no difference. Gruenberg (1964) raised the question of whether or not mildly retarded individuals who disappear from services after leaving school are indistinguishable from others in their daily lives. Of all individuals with MR, it is they who most strive to pass as "normal" (Edgerton, 1967). Atypical appearance may be a social obstacle.

We found that subjects with mild MR who received no adult mental retardation services were significantly more atypical in appearance than their matched comparisons ($t[69] = 4.64, p < .001$. This difference should be considered, however, in conjunction with the finding that 29 percent of these young adults with mild MR showed no evidence of atypical appearance, and a further 30 percent showed only one mild atypicality. The statistical difference found between the matched pairs should not lead to the assumption that all or most of the young adults with mild MR who received no adult mental retardation services appeared atypical.

We have already shown that atypical appearance increased with severity of mental retardation, so all the other subsets of the population with MR would also have significant and increasingly greater differences from the comparisons.

The descriptions of atypical appearance classified under a particular component can be instructive in trying to reduce atypicality and indicate whether the atypicality gives clues that a person has MR. Atypical expression/manner is a component in which various forms of behavior are likely to be involved. Content analysis of this component suggested three categories: eye behavior only, facial expressions not including eyes, and hand and arm movement. Because atypical expression and manner was one of two components that appeared with any frequency among comparisons, the subjects with mild MR who received no adult mental retardation services were contrasted with comparisons on these categories within that component. The main difference was in eye behavior, which was noted for 28 percent of the subjects with mild MR who had an atypical expression or manner and was not found among comparisons. Examples of expression and manner that were coded from descriptions of the eyes were "often closed left eye and looked at interviewer with right eye only," "eyes dull and slow-moving," "did not look at interviewer directly very often," "stared at interviewer." Because these examples of eye behavior were unique to the young people with mild MR, they may give cues of intellectual limitations, and it might be useful to consider whether they could be changed. An analysis of the content of all the components is beyond our scope in this chapter, but the illustrations suggest that the issue is worth further investigation.

Summary and Conclusions

The research evidence showing that appearance influences social relations, the development of self-image, and the socialization process led us to believe that appearance is a salient variable that should be included in the study of people with mental retardation. No summary measure of appearance that includes dynamic as well as static components is available, so we made a first attempt to develop such a measure. The measure has some validity because hypotheses based on theory were confirmed. We recognize that careful testing should have been carried out on the reliability of the interviewers' observations of appearance, but having two observers for even a sample of subjects was beyond our resources, and we wanted to take advantage of the unusual opportunity of having some measure of appearance for a total population of young adults with MR and comparison subjects. It is reasonable to expect that trained observers will have some degree of reliability, but studies of interpersonal perception are needed.

Several issues related to the measure that we developed need study. First, implicit in the measure is the assumption that those with the same summary score are comparable in the responses that they will elicit from others. It is not clear, however, whether people will respond in a similar way to a man who is obese (rated 3) and ugly (rated 3) and to someone with several different slight and moderate components of atypicality but the same summary rating of 6. Second, we do not know whether the violation of expectation increases in a linear manner across the range of the summary measure or whether reactions might shift abruptly at certain points in the scale. Finally, two important factors were omitted from this appearance measure: characteristics amenable to change (for instance, dress, grooming, and cleanliness) and characteristics that elicit a positive response and facilitate social intercourse (such as grace, coordinated movement, and a ready, pleasant smile). These characteristics may mitigate or even offset the consequences of the components of appearance that we selected. We did not include these characteristics because they might have changed over the time period in which we were interested.

Contrary to the expectation of Tarjan (1970) that individuals with MR who disappear from services after leaving school are indistinguishable from nonretarded peers, our results suggest that as a group, these adults are more atypical in appearance. Individually, however, many probably are indistinguishable.

The importance of appearance as a clue to understanding individuals and interpersonal behavior has long been recognized in literature and drama, and more recently by behavioral scientists. The clear power and importance of appearance variables are good reasons for their development and use in research.

13

Self-Esteem

The variables dealing with personal characteristics that have been described thus far were based on the assessments and observations of others. In Chapter 4, we indicated that an important part of the follow-up study design was to learn about the thoughts and feelings of the young people being studied. In this chapter, we will use a measure of self-esteem based on their responses to questions designed to elicit information about how they felt about themselves (see Facchini 1995).

In general, the ways in which we conduct ourselves are influenced by how others perceive us and behave toward us. It is likely that individuals with mental retardation (MR) experience disparaging behavior from others at some time. They are also generally aware that, in some ways, they are less competent than most other people. Behavior toward those with MR is likely to be influenced by direct observation of their incompetence and by the values and stereotypes about MR that may be prevalent in the society. For these reasons, it is likely that individuals with MR will, in general, have lower self-esteem than peers who do not have MR. Throughout this book, it becomes apparent that the personal characteristics and histories of young people with MR are heterogeneous, and that we may expect wide variation in levels of self-esteem as a result.

In this chapter, we will compare the level of self-esteem of two groups of young adults: those with mild MR and peers who did not have MR who were selected as a comparison population for the present study. We will also determine what personal characteristics and histories of the young people with MR were related to different levels of self-esteem.

The self-esteem measure was influenced by Harter's (1982) conceptualization of "perceived competence." Among children with low IQ's, Harter found that three dimensions of perceived competence emerged: cognitive, social, and general. These dimensions appeared relevant for the young adults in the present study and were used as a guide in selecting questions from the interview that were related to self-esteem. These dealt with schooling, employment, social relationships, spare time activities, and some questions of a more general nature. A total of ninety-two questions in which informants could express feelings about themselves were used.

Questions about school asked for information on how the informants felt when they first went there, whether they had friends at school, and if not, why not. If the young people reported being teased, bullied, treated unfairly, or left out of things, explanations were sought.

Questions about jobs included what individuals liked and disliked about their present job, how they got along with various people at work, and about their working life in general, such as whether there was other work they would have preferred. As with their school experiences, if they reported ever having been teased, bullied, or treated unfairly in their work histories, they were asked for explanations of the experiences.

More general questions asked how well they got along with other people and whether they had any difficulties making friends with members of either sex, whether they were shy, lost their temper easily, and got into fights, and whether there were things they wished they could do but were unable to. They were also asked to conjecture about what the next ten years might hold for them, including problems they might have and their hopes for the future.

Each response that was judged to include a self-evaluation statement was coded on a scale indicating whether the self-evaluation was positive, neutral, mixed, or negative. From all these (except neutral responses, which were omitted), we developed a composite measure of self-esteem.

Finally, after having coded the above items, the coder made a subjective judgment in response to the question, "In general, what does this individual think of him/herself?" The coder then rated the individual's self-esteem on a 5-point scale (1 = worthless to 5 = very good).

A more complete description of the methods is given in Facchini (1995), which includes analyses of subscales for the different dimensions, and analyses of reliability and validity based on a 10 percent random independent double coding. Acceptable reliability and validity were obtained for both the objective and subjective measures. The composite measure, based on the objective rating from all the dimensions, was compared with the subjective measure, and there was high agreement. The analysis was restricted to those who were able to give the responses needed for examination of self-esteem. All the young adults with severe MR, and a few of those with mild MR, were unable to give the needed responses. The following results are based on the subjective measure.

The mean self-esteem ratings for those with mild MR and the non-retarded comparisons are shown in Table 13.1. A *t*-test indicated that the young adults with mild MR had significantly lower self-esteem than did the comparisons.

To consider what factors may be related to level of self-esteem, the remainder of the analysis will focus exclusively on young adults with mild MR. Some analyses were done for males and females separately, and some for them combined.

Family

In Chapters 6 and 14 we examine the family environments experienced by the young people with MR during their upbringing and in Chapter 8, the influence of family stability on their behavior. Because

Table 13.1 Mean self-esteem ratings for young adults with mild mental retardation and comparison population

Group	*N*	Mean[a]	SD	Median
Mild MR	86	3.08	1.4	3.0
Comparisons	91	4.23	1.0	5.0

a. Scores were on a 5-point scale: 1 = worthless, 5 = very good.

of these findings, we expected that young adults who had unstable family histories would have lower self-esteem than those who had stable histories. Using Pearson correlations, we confirmed this expectation for the group as a whole ($r = -.239$, $p < .01$) as well as for females ($r = -.312$, $p < .02$). The relationship was weaker for males ($r = -.184$, $p < .10$), a gender difference due perhaps to the closer ties the young women maintained with their families than did the young men.

Social Interaction with Peers

Young adults' frequent social interaction with peers may be related to self-esteem in two ways: socializing frequently with peers may indicate high self-esteem; high self-esteem may also be, in part, the result of having been successful in peer relationships and of having some social skills. A measure of social interaction is described in Chapter 17. It was made up of the three categories of amount of time spent socializing with peers. No gender differences were found in the relationship between social interaction and self-esteem. For males and females combined, analysis of variance was significant. A subsequent Least Significant Difference procedure showed that young adults whose social interactions were frequent and seldom had significantly higher self-esteem than those who reported none. There was no significant difference between the self-esteem of those whose social interaction was frequent and those whose social interaction was seldom (see Table 13.2). This provides partial confirmation of our expectation.

Adult Behavior Disturbance

Some forms of behavior disturbance in young adults are likely to both lead to, and be a consequence of, a lower level of self-esteem (see Chapter 8 for definitions of the behavior disturbance measures). A separate correlational analysis was carried out for males and for females. No significant relationship was found between the overall measure of behavior disturbance and self-esteem, but there were some for components of the behavior disturbance ratings. For males, lower self-esteem was related to emotional disturbance ($r = -.239$, $p < .04$) and aggressive conduct disorder ($r = -.234$, $p < .04$). For

Table 13.2 Mean self-esteem ratings for young adults with mild mental retardation by frequency of socializing with peers

Socialized with peers	*N*	Mean	SD
Frequently	54	3.31	1.16
Seldom	18	3.44	1.25
Not at all	24	2.33	1.30

females, lower self-esteem was related to aggressive conduct disorder ($r = -.312$, $p < .025$) and antisocial behavior ($r = -.309$, $p < .025$); there was close to a significant relationship with emotional disturbance ($r = -.243$, $p < .06$).

Job History

Chapter 16 gives measures related to job history and defines level of job skill. We expected that young adults who held jobs requiring more skill would have higher self-esteem than those in jobs requiring less skill. We did not obtain the expected result, possibly because all the young adults with MR had jobs at the low end of the scale of job skills, either semiskilled or unskilled manual work, both of which are less generally esteemed by the community than jobs requiring higher levels of skill. An experience related to job histories that may have a greater association with level of self-esteem than the distinction between semi-skilled and unskilled jobs is how much time the young adult is unemployed and seeking employment. We found that young adults with high rates of unemployment had lower self-esteem than those with little or no unemployment between the time they left school and age 22 ($r = -.282$, $p < .05$).

Marriage

Marriage confers a status that is more generally approved by society than remaining single and thus may help a person's self-esteem. Among those with mild MR, individuals who married were among the more able, especially the men (see Chapter 17). We expected then, that those who were married would have higher self-esteem than those who remained single. The results confirmed this expectation. Analysis of variance showed that young adults who were married or cohabiting (combined) had a significantly ($p < .05$) higher mean self-esteem rating ($n = 25$, mean = 3.52, SD = 1.19) than those who were single ($n = 70$, mean = 2.86, SD = 1.34).

We examined some additional factors that might be related to self-esteem—IQ within the mild MR range, childhood behavior disturbance, and school placement history—but these did not turn out to be significant.

Relative Importance of Factors Related to Self-Esteem

To determine the relative importance of the variables shown to be related to self-esteem, we carried out a stepwise multiple regression for males and females combined. Only marital status, peer social interactions, and aggressive conduct disorders were found to contribute significantly to the variance on self-esteem. Family stability, unemployment, and the other types of behavior disturbance were not found to make significant contributions in the context of the other variables. The final model accounted for 26 percent of the variance.

Summary and Conclusions

The results confirmed some, but not all, of our expectations. Young adults with mild MR had lower self-esteem than the nonretarded comparisons. Among those with mild MR, family stability was the only measure of childhood experience to show some relationship to self-esteem, but its importance was diminished in the presence of other variables when a multiple regression analysis was carried out. The adult variables, socializing with peers and marital status, were both shown to be related to self-esteem. It is probable that young people with good self-esteem are able to develop and keep social relationships. At the same time, good social relationships may bolster self-esteem.

Among the types of adult behavior disturbance, only aggressive conduct disorder was strongly related to self-esteem for both males and females. It may be that aggression is a response to feelings of inadequacy. It was of some interest that, while antisocial behavior was more common among males than females (see Chapter 8), it was only related to self-esteem for females. A finding that antisocial behavior also occurred with some frequency among comparison males but was nonexistent among comparison females may help to explain this finding . Perhaps, for the young men with MR, antisocial behavior elevated their status among peers somewhat, whereas, for the young women, it diminished their status. It must be recalled that almost none of the antisocial behavior was of a very serious nature.

Part IV

Histories

14

Upbringing and Family Histories

The primary influences on the social, intellectual and emotional development of children are the adults responsible for their upbringing. For most children, the biological parents serve this role. But some children, because of parental death, family break-up, or other reasons such as abandonment, neglect, or abuse, must be placed with substitute caretakers, who may be relatives, friends of the parents, foster or adoptive parents, or people in charge of various homes and institutions responsible for the care of the resident children. From the histories of the children in the follow-up study we learned that many were not cared for consistently by their biological parents, and that some who did live with biological parents experienced abuse, neglect, poverty, and severe parental discord. As we discovered, we needed ways to describe the children's histories that would take into account all the various kinds of upbringing they had experienced. There is no single term to characterize this diversity, and we found it necessary to stretch the definition of "family" to include the various possibilities we have briefly described. Despite the large body of research devoted to the family, we could find no single definition that encompassed the diversity in the study population. Turnbull, Summers, and Brotherson (1986) reached a similar conclusion: "A major gap in family systems and mental retardation literature is an operational definition of a family" (p. 46).

To develop a picture of the children's family histories, we will use three measures: social class, family stability, and family groupings based on a cluster analysis. We will examine these three measures separately, and in combination, in order to determine the variability in the families of the children with mental retardation (MR) and how similar or different they were from the families of the comparison group. Finally, we will look at both the extent and the kinds of substitute caretaking the children received and provide brief descriptions of the children with MR and their families.

Social Class

Social class provides a general indicator of family lifestyle. The classification used here was based on the British Registrar General's scheme (British Register Office 1951), in which the occupations of the heads of households that were roughly comparable in economic and social terms were divided into five categories, ranging from Social Class I (Professional) to Social Class V (Unskilled manual laborer). In the initial Aberdeen study of mental retardation (see Birch et al. 1970; Chapter 1), Social Class III (Skilled Workers) was found to encompass half the population. To obtain social class groupings more equal in size, Social Class III was subdivided and reorganized as follows: I–IIIa, Nonmanual; IIIb, Journeyman and artisan; IIIc, Other skilled manual; IV, Semiskilled manual; V Unskilled manual.

A similar concept, "socioeconomic status," based on occupation, education, and income, has been used in the United States. Studies in Aberdeen, however, showed that income and education were so closely related to occupation that occupation alone could be used.

The use of social class for the follow-up study presents both advantages and disadvantages. It is relatively easy to obtain information from a family about the occupation of the head of the household; for our study, the measure had been obtained for a one-in-five random sample of all children in Aberdeen in the birth cohorts we were studying. At the same time, this classification is based on a premise that does not hold for some families; that is, that there is a head of the household who has a job or a job history. We needed a family classification that covered not merely one point in time but the entire time span of childhood, and the premise becomes weaker the longer the time span. Despite its limitations, this classification was useful for the majority of families. For the children whose families did not fit the classification, we added the category "not classifiable." (For additional discussion of social class, see Chapter 1 on the initial study and Chapter 5 dealing with prevalence. Social class was also used as a matching variable in the selection of comparisons; see Chapter 4 on design and methods.)

Family Stability

Because social class provides no indication of family dynamics or changes during a child's upbringing, we developed a family stability measure with a five-point scale that ranged from 1, stable family environment, in which the child lived throughout with both parents and there was no evidence of family dysfunction or pathology, to 5, markedly unstable environment, in which the child experienced family disorganization, disruptions, and discord, and often a series of caretakers. For a full description of the scale, see Richardson, Koller, and Katz (1985a) and Chapter 5, where it was used as an indicator of psychosocial adversity. The measure provides some indication of the child's history in the family context.

Family Clusters

We needed a third family measure that would provide additional information about the histories of the children's caretakers. In most cases, these were the biological parents, but if the child was adopted, fostered, or cared for by a relative for most of his or her upbringing, these substitute parents were included in the cluster analysis. We did not assume that all children lived consistently with their parents. For example, if the child was placed in an institution, we included the histories of the child's parents in the classification as long as they maintained contact with the child.

The first step in the cluster analysis was to select variables that described aspects of the father's and mother's histories, and general variables that described family functioning. In all, we selected twenty-eight variables and subjected them to factor analyses using the families of both the children with MR and the comparisons. The factor analyses yielded ten factors. For each parent, there were factors describing disabilities, chronic illness, and psychiatric illness. The remaining factors dealt with parents' criminal behavior, parents' intellectual limitations, family disharmony and changes in the household, number of children and social class, and deaths of siblings of the study child.

Using the ten factor scores, we performed a cluster analysis using 177 families of children with MR and 172 families of comparisons. (A complete description of the methods and the validation procedures, along with a description of each cluster, may be found in Koller, Richardson, and Katz 1992.) The procedure draws families together into relatively homogeneous groups based on their similarities across the factor scores. The resulting twenty-four different clusters indicate the heterogeneity of the families in the study. The clusters ranged in size from 1 to 56 families, and thirteen clusters had 6 or more.

While each cluster was different from every other, we were able to group them according to the amount and types of family dysfunction or adversity present. We placed twenty-one of the twenty-four clusters into four general categories related to family adversity: No evidence of adversity; Parent(s) with chronic disabilities or illness; Parent(s) with psychiatric illness; Multiple adversity with ill health and/or psychiatric illness combined with general family adversity. This included parents with criminal behavior, intellectual limitation, family disharmony, changes in the household, large numbers of children, and childhood deaths in the family. The three remaining clusters did not fit into these categories. These were cluster L, high scores on death of children; cluster I, high scores on death of children and parents with limited intelligence, family disharmony and disruption, and changes in the family; and cluster E, which included families with parents of limited intelligence, family disharmony, and changes in the family.

Finally, some families were omitted from the cluster analysis because of missing information or because they were so unusual they did not have histories relevant to the variables used in the cluster analysis.

Comparing the Families of Children with MR and Comparisons

Social Class

Because social class was used as a matching variable in the selection of comparisons for the study, we could not use the comparisons in this analysis. In Chapter 5 we showed that there was no difference between the social class distribution of the families of children with severe MR and the families of children in the community who did not have MR; however, the families of children with mild MR were found, far more frequently than the general population of families in Aberdeen, at the lower end of the social class scale.

Family Stability

The families of children with mental retardation were markedly more unstable than the families of the comparisons (see Table 14.1). We carried out other analyses of the family stability measure, which showed that families who were rated 3 to 5 on the scale (less stable) were distinct from families who were rated 1 and 2 on the scale (more stable) (Richardson, Koller, and Katz 1985a). Forty-five percent of the families of the children with MR but less than 6 percent of the comparisons were at the more unstable end of the scale.

Family Clusters

There were some differences between families of children with MR and the comparison families whose children were not MR (see Table 14.2). In the group of clusters where there was no evidence of family adversity, there were more comparison families (54 percent) than families with a child with MR (33 percent). Cluster 5 did not fit into the four cluster groupings and was characterized by high scores on deaths of children in the family. This cluster was more frequent for

Table 14.1 Family stability of matched pairs of children with mental retardation and comparisons (in percent)

	Children with MR	Comparison children
1. Stable family	28	59
2. Continuous care	27	36
3. Stressful family	27	5
4. Disorganized family	8	<1
5. Markedly unstable	10	0
Total *N*	143	143

Table 14.2 Groups of clusters and percentages of families with children with mental retardation and comparisons

Forms of adversity	Clusters[a]	Families: Of children with MR	Families: Of comparisons
Cluster Groups			
1. No evidence of adversity	C,J,A	33	54
2. Parent(s) chronic disability or illness	M,K,B,S,D	17	21
3. Parent(s) psychiatric illness	F,H,V,G	8	6
4. Parent(s) ill health and/or psychiatric illness and other adversity	X,N,U,P, Q,W,R,T,O	11	1
Single Clusters			
5. High score on deaths of children	L	12	8
6. Limited parent intelligence, family discord and change, high score on child deaths	I	3	<1
7. Parents with limited intelligence, family disharmony, and changes in the family	E	4	5
Families not included because of missing information or unusual histories		12	4
Total number of families		177[b]	172

a. Letters refer to clusters shown in Koller et al. 1992.
b. Because fourteen families had more than one child in the study with MR, the number of families is smaller than the number of children.

families of children with MR (12 percent) than for families of comparisons (8 percent). For the two remaining clusters (6 and 7), no noticeable differences were found.

Placement in Care

We wanted to find out whether the children with MR in our study were more often placed in foster care, or in residences run by the local authorities or voluntary agencies, than either the comparison children or all other children in the city who did not have MR. The Children's Department provided us with a census of all the children in their care on March 1, 1964, who had been born between 1951 and 1955, the birth cohorts of the children in the present study. At the time of the census, the study children ranged in age from 9 to

13 years. The census indicated whether placement was in foster care or in a children's residence. These residences were open to all children in need, and were not intended for children with MR in particular.

The children with MR from our study were in foster care three times as often as all other Aberdeen children (1.8 percent and 0.56 percent, respectively), while no comparison children were in foster care. In addition, more children with MR were in residences than either comparisons or all other children in the city who did not have MR (3.6 percent, 0.58 percent, 0.55 percent, respectively). The percentage of children with MR in children's homes was, then, over six times higher than the percentages in the other two groups that did not have MR. The figures from the census, which are for one particular day, would clearly be higher if the census had been for the whole period of childhood.

Thus, the families of children with both mild and severe MR differed from others in the following ways:

1. Families of children with mild MR were more frequently found at the lower end of the social class scale, but this difference was not evident for families of children with severe MR.
2. They were more frequently unstable.
3. They were more frequently in clusters where there was multiple adversity, and less frequently in clusters where there was an absence of adversity.
4. They more frequently had histories that were so atypical, they did not fit the variables in the cluster analysis.
5. The children with MR more often lived with foster parents or in a children's home run by the local authorities or by voluntary agencies.

Families of Children with Mental Retardation

Thus far we have examined each of the measures dealing with families, contrasting families who had children with MR with those who did not. Here we will narrow the focus to the families that most interest us: those who had children with MR. For these families, we will examine the association between social class and family stability, and then the families described in the cluster analysis in the context of these two factors.

Social Class and Family Stability

For families of children with mental retardation, social class and family stability were significantly related: a larger percentage of children from unstable families (3–5 on the scale) came from the lower social classes (see Table 14.3). Two thirds of all the families were stable (1–2 on the scale). It is important to note that stable families were found in all social classes with similar frequency, whereas the percentage of unstable families increased in a stepwise manner from upper to lower social class, with the largest percentage, by far, found in social class V. It is not shown on Table 14.3, but the "unclassified" families, who could not be assigned a social class, were all unstable.

Family Custers

Using all three of the measures together provides the most comprehensive view of the families of children with MR. Table 14.4 shows the family clusters, and those not included in the cluster analysis, in the context of social class and family stability. On conceptual grounds, we anticipated that the four groups of family clusters shown in Table 14.4 would have different distributions of social class and family stability. As the amount and kinds of family adversity increased, as shown in the cluster groups, we anticipated that there would be increasing proportions of families that were unstable and toward the lower end of the social class scale, including those not classifiable. In Table 14.4, where the family cluster groups are ranked from least adversity to most adversity, the distribution of social class and family stability for each cluster group confirms these expectations. In the group with no evidence of family adversity, the percentages varied little across

Table 14.3 Percentages of families with children with mental retardation by social class and family stability

Family stability[a]	Social class					*N*
	I–IIIa	IIIb	IIIc	IV	V	
1–2	17	21	22	16	23	112
3–5	8	11	14	21	46	63

a. See Table 14.1 for definitions.

Table 14.4 Social class and family stability of the family clusters and families excluded from the cluster analysis in families of children with mental retardation (in percent)

Forms of adversity	Social class							
	I–IIIa	IIIb	IIIc	IV	V	Not classifiable	Family Stability 3–5	*N*
Cluster Groups[a]								
1. No evidence	19	24	20	20	17	0	7	59
2. Parent chronic disability and illness	17	20	13	17	27	7	30	30
3. Parent psychiatric illness	13	20	7	13	33	13	80	15
4. Multiple adversity	0	0	11	11	41	47	94	19
Single Clusters								
5. High score on death of child	5	10	24	14	48	0	24	21
6. High score on child death and limited parent intelligence, family discord, and changes in household	0	0	33	33	17	17	67	6
7. Limited parent intelligence, family disharmony, and changes in household	29	14	29	0	14	14	58	7
Families that could not be placed in clusters	10	10	10	14	29	29	76	21

a. See Table 14.2 for clusters that made up the groups.

the social class scale, all could be assigned a social class, and this group had the lowest percentage of unstable families of any of the four. The heaviest overrepresentation at the low end of the social class scale was in the cluster group with multiple family adversity; this group had the largest percentage not classifiable and virtually all (94 percent) were unstable families. In the two intermediate groups of parent chronic disability and illness, and parent psychiatric illness, the social class distributions were similar, but the families with psychiatric illness less often could be assigned a social class and were unstable twice as often as families with chronic disability and illness.

The variables that define clusters 6 and 7 indicate that there was some adversity in the upbringing of the children, and this is also indicated by the high proportion of family instability in these clusters. Cluster 5 was outstanding only in deaths of children. This may have been related to biological or social factors and, if biological, provides no conceptual link with social class or family stability. It may be expected that clusters 6 and 7 would have more unstable families than cluster 5 and more families that could not be assigned a social class, and these expectations were confirmed.

Frequency and Kinds of Substitute Parents

The clusters were based largely on the histories of the parents or parent substitutes and gave no indication of whether their children with MR lived with them consistently or not. We have already given some information about the history of caretakers for children in the families who would not fit into the clusters. The following is a summary of the upbringing of the children with MR who were included in the clusters:

Seventy percent lived with their biological parents throughout their childhood.

Eleven percent were in some form of institutional care where they remained twenty-four hours a day. Three-quarters of these children were in institutions for children with mental retardation. The remainder were in institutions for psychiatric care, with the exception of one who was in an institution for those with epilepsy.

Eleven percent did not live with parents but were in various kinds of residences, and attended special educational facilities for children with mental retardation during the day.

Four percent lived with grandparent(s).

Four percent were raised by a single foster family or were adopted.

Twenty-one families were not included in the cluster analysis, some because of lack of information and some because the children did not live with their parents. Three children were abandoned and placed in mental retardation institutions early in life and remained there until adulthood. Six children, because of parental death, divorce, or separation, or because of neglect, abandonment, or abuse, spent their childhood in the care of the city's Children's Department, and were placed in foster care or in residences run either by the city or by voluntary agencies. Most of those children had several different placements during childhood.

The following histories of children with MR and their families illustrate the different cluster groups and families that could not be placed in clusters.

Cluster Group, No Evidence of Adversity. Social Class IIIb. Family Stability 1

Ann's parents had both been brought up in Aberdeen but after their marriage had moved to Wales, where her father took a job in the town transport department supervising the repair of buses. They had two daughters, and Ann was the second. There was nothing unusual about her appearance, and it took some time before it became apparent that she was developing more slowly than other children. At the beginning, Ann's parents were not particularly concerned because they knew that children develop at different rates, but she did not walk properly until she was nearly four. She had problems with her feet and eyes and was under medical care. When she went to the local primary school, it soon became apparent that she could not cope with schoolwork. The headmaster told her mother that Ann had mental retardation, something her mother had not faced up to. Ann's parents knew that Aberdeen had a very good hospital and school system, and since the special education facilities where they lived were not good, they decided to move there so that Ann might get better help.

Ann was placed in the special school and seemed happy there. She was easy to get along with and had a cheerful, good-natured disposition. Although she was popular with the other children at the school, she had no friends in the neighborhood where she lived. Most of the neighbors were very kind to her, but a few children teased her about going to the special school. Ann's older sister was a great support to her, her father joined in the children's activities when they were home, and the family went on holidays together. Her parents had always hoped somehow that something would happen so that Ann would be able to lead a more normal life. They did not discuss this because it was so upsetting, but they knew in their hearts that the problems with Ann would always be there.

Later in her schooling, Ann's father was transferred to a job in a rural area. The local education authorities arranged for Ann to attend a residential school for children with mental retardation. The school was near the home of a relative, who frequently visited Ann at the school. Ann's parents and sister also visited, and would take her out on excursions and home at weekends. At the age of 16, Ann had to leave the special residential school, and she returned home to live with her family. Throughout her childhood, Ann's relatives had always been accepting of her disability and very supportive of her and her family.

Cluster Group, No Evidence of Adversity. Social Class I–IIIa. Family Stability 2

John was an only child, and his parents lived in the same house throughout his upbringing. His father worked as a government administrator, and his mother was a housewife. John developed very slowly and was unable to speak in sentences until he was four. From an early age, John's behavior was very disturbed. He was highly nervous and excitable, impulsive and restless. When his mother took him downtown shopping, he would lie down in the street and have temper tantrums, and she would be unable to manage him. Finally she had to stop taking him shopping. She was also unable to visit friends and relatives because of John's behavior. As a result of the stress of looking after John, both parents became exhausted and his mother became depressed. When they went on holidays, they could not stay at hotels or bed and breakfast facilities because of John's behavior, so they went on caravan (camping) holidays. At age eight, John was expelled from the special school because he needed constant supervision and an inordinate amount of teacher time. His hyperactivity caused problems both in the classroom and on the playground. When his mother came to take him home from school, he would run away. She was on the verge of a breakdown, and it was arranged for John to be placed in a residential home to give his parents some respite. They used the respite to go on holiday, but were so exhausted that all they could do was just sit. John's father found it difficult to relate to him, and this, combined with the overall stress, caused the marital relationship to suffer. After the respite care, it was decided that John should be placed permanently in an institution. John's parents visited him there and sometimes took him home for a short visit, but because of his continued disturbed behavior, they dreaded these occasions.

In both families, the parents lived together during the upbringing of the child. John, however, was a greater source of stress to his parents than Ann was to hers. In forming the clusters, we did not take the "child as the source of stress" into account. John's parents experienced some difficulties in their marital relationship, which is shown in a rating of 2 in family stability, compared to a rating of 1 for Ann's parents, who showed no evidence of marital problems.

Cluster Group, Parent Chronic Disability and Illness. Social Class, Not Classifiable. Family Stability 3

David was the fourth of seven children. His father had been unemployed throughout his childhood because of wounds suffered during the war and severe asthma, and he had been hospitalized on several occasions. David's mother was a housewife. The family had lived in a series of small, crowded, rented flats, and their income came from social security and a wartime disability pension. Two of the children lived with their grandparents, who later adopted them. When David was eight, the family was evicted from their flat for rent arrears. They were taken in by one of David's aunts, and there followed a series of makeshift, unsatisfactory housing arrangements, with increasing marital disharmony. Eventually they obtained a house, where they were able to remain. David attended regular schools until age eight, when he was transferred to the special school. He had previously been given remedial instruction, but his writing and spelling were so poor that the transfer was deemed advisable. Before the transfer, David appeared to be high strung and nervous, but after going to the special school, he became calmer and more relaxed. David reported that he felt really wanted at the special school and that the teachers were very good to him. His school reports described him as pleasant, hardworking, and well-behaved. There were also references to his being poorly clad and lacking in cleanliness.

David's father had a chronic disability. The poor housing, low income, their eviction and living arrangements were not variables included in the factor analysis, but the lack of a wage-earner is indicated by the unclassifiable social class. The disharmony between parents who continued to live together, combined with a period when there were housing problems, is indicated by the family stability score of 3, which places the family in the unstable group (3–5).

Cluster Group, Parent Psychiatric Illness. Social Class, Not Classifiable. Family Stability 5

Kathleen's father met his future wife when he was in the army in Germany after World War II. She was a concentration camp survivor and had had a terrible early life. Kathleen's parents had two sons while they were in Germany and then returned to Aberdeen, Kathleen's father's birthplace. Kathleen was born several years later. The family was forced to move twice when their house was condemned by the local authorities as unfit for human habitation. Kathleen's mother suffered from psychiatric problems. Her parents did not get along and only stayed together for the sake of the children. They received no help with their problems from relatives, but their neighbors were always kindly. When Kathleen was two years old, her mother entered a psychiatric hospital; from then on, she was in and out of the hospital and spent more time there than at home. Because of family problems, Kathleen was placed in a residential nursery and then for a year in the care of a woman who took in foster children. The conditions in this woman's home were so bad that the neighbors complained, and Kathleen was moved to a residence run by the local authorities, where her brothers had already been placed. Between ages 4 and 14, Kathleen lived in four different residences, with periods at home when her mother was out of the hospital. On one occasion, she was taken into care because her mother said she was unmanageable.

Kathleen's education began at a regular school, where she remained until she was 9. She was then transferred to the special school for children with MR. As the school transfer records reported, "Class work is very below standard. Behavior irresponsible. Does not respond to training." The very poor home conditions were noted.

During her early years in local authority residences, Kathleen was very unhappy, but as she grew older she got to like them. Her father visited her every week or so, and her mother when she was able. They used to bring her dog, to which she was deeply attached. Kathleen's father developed health problems when she was 12 years old and died a year later. For her last two years of school, Kathleen was able to live at home with her mother, who by now was doing better. The records of her early years at the special school indicated little progress in class work and some problems in behavior, as evidenced by remarks such as "restless, inattentive, quite a nuisance." As she grew older, her class work improved, and positive comments became more frequent: "very lively, very interested in the world around her, unquashable."

Cluster Group, Multiple Adversity. Social Class Not Classifiable. Family Stability 5

James was the third of six children. For the first eight years of his life, he lived with his mother and father, but his father was often away from home. His father had rarely worked. He was a heavy drinker, frequently fought with his wife, and sometimes battered her. At times, he would go with other women. He got into trouble with the law and spent time in jail. Once he sold all the furniture and left the family with an empty house. James's brother recalled that the times his father was in jail were the happiest years of their childhood. The family was extremely poor, and for a time the mother worked, but she soon found it too difficult in addition to coping with her husband and the children. She wanted to leave her husband but would not leave the children. Because of the conflict in the house, the oldest child went to live with her grandmother.

When James was ten years old, his mother died suddenly. The cause was not clear but may have been suicide. His sister described the effect of her death on James: "He was always the one that needed that extra bit of attention, and he missed it. There was no sort of love left for the family. He just didn't have anything to hang on to anymore." After his mother died, James's father was on the verge of a mental breakdown, and he received treatment at a psychiatric clinic. The family was evicted from their home for not paying rent, and James went to stay with an aunt. His father was drinking and often left the children on their own. He was unable to cope with the children and placed them in a local authority residence. When James was 12, his father remarried, brought the children home, and shortly afterwards moved to be near his brother in England.

James had attended a regular school in Aberdeen until age 8. Then he was transferred to the special school, where he remained until he went with the family to England. His school reports indicated that James was well-behaved and pleasant, had no problems, and was doing well in his schoolwork. While in England, James first attended a special school, but his father took him out and placed him in a regular school. After a year, the family moved back to Aberdeen and James returned to the special school. His stepmother was described as having no affection for the children, and she and James's father both drank heavily. They were not able to cope with the children but would not relinquish their care to their grandmother. Instead, they placed the children in a local authority residence. Shortly afterwards, the Children's Department of the city took over their care, acting in part on reports from the National Society for the Prevention of Cruelty to Children. James spent the remainder of his childhood in several different local authority residences.

After his return to Aberdeen from England, James's school reports showed that he had developed behavior problems. These eventually became so severe that James was sent to a residential institution for persons with mental retardation and psychiatric problems.

Each of the families thus far described belonged to one of the four groups of clusters. But 23 children were not included in the family clusters because the data were insufficient. The following cases indicate some of the reasons why they had to be omitted.

Social Class Not Classifiable. Family Stability 5

Don was one of ten children. The family lived in appalling conditions. He was so poorly fed that, when taken to the hospital as an infant, the staff recorded that he had marasmus, or chronic malnutrition. When Don was 1 year old the Home Health Visitor noted, "Neglected, but no external evidence of cruelty. Dirty both scalp and body. Flea bites. Home and child dirty and smelly." She also noted that all the children were incontinent. Don lived with his family until he was 13. At age 8, he was transferred from a regular school to the special school for children with mental retardation. He had been making very poor educational progress, and it was noted that his home conditions were unsatisfactory, with severe overcrowding. He was described as emotionally disturbed, incontinent, solitary, and timid. At age 9, it was noted that he had lice in his hair, and he was temporarily suspended from school at age 13 because of lice. Don ran away from home several times. The family was a source of concern to the social work department, and the father was given a home help aide to try to improve the conditions at home. According to Don, his mother sat around and gave no help when the home help aide was at the house. Don's father was an unskilled laborer and often unemployed. He drank heavily and spent time in prison for stealing. Conditions in the home became so bad that Don and all his siblings were removed from their parents and placed in local authority children's residences. Don was 18 years old when his father died. His mother would not agree to be interviewed for the follow-up study.

Social Class Not Classifiable. Family Stability 5

Molly was placed in a residential nursery when she was two months old. There is very little information about her parents. One source indicated that both were killed in a car crash, another that they were divorced before Molly was conceived and that she was abandoned by her mother. Whatever happened, the parents were never traced. At age two, Molly was looked after by a foster mother for six months and then lived in a series of residential homes for children until age 18, when she moved into lodgings approved by the local authorities.

15

Paths through Mental Retardation Services

In Chapter 5, on prevalence, we showed the number of individuals with mental retardation (MR) in any type of MR service at each age from 5 to 22 years. This age perspective is useful in estimating service needs for groups within the total population of young people with MR.

In the present chapter, however, we will look at MR services from a different perspective. We will trace each individual's path through these services and examine the factors that influenced their placement by considering the interaction of the personal characteristics of the young people, their family backgrounds, and the policies and practices of various local authorities in Aberdeen.

MR services for children were separate from those for adults, the transition between them occurring around 15 or 16 years of age. We will focus first on children's services, and then on adult services and their links with the childhood paths.

Children's Histories in Mental Retardation Services

Table 15.1 shows the initial placement of each child in mental retardation services (column 1) and the paths to final placements upon leaving school (column 2). The personal characteristics of the children in each path are shown in columns 3–10, followed by the children's family stability and the number who died in each path. To aid in understanding the paths, we will first describe the various MR services available to children.

MR Services for Children

Day services. The day services for children with MR were under the jurisdiction of the local education authorities, who laid the original plans for these services in the 1950s, when generally negative stereotypes about children with MR prevailed. The planners were well aware of, and often shared, contemporary community values, and this influenced their decisions. They concluded that the interests of children with MR would be best served by providing services in separate facilities away from other children, either in a special school or, for those who were deemed unable to benefit from the curriculum there, in a Junior Occupation Center (JOC).

The educational services planners built the special school on a large and attractive site in an upper-income area of the city in order to provide an advantageous physical environment. Class sizes were smaller than in the regular schools. Selected teachers, with competence and experience in regular schools, were sent for two years of training in special education, paid a full salary while training, and then given salaries higher than teachers in regular schools. When the special school was planned, it was envisioned as serving children in the area surrounding Aberdeen as well as in the city itself.

During construction, however, the educational authorities in the surrounding areas decided not to use the new special school in Aberdeen. As a result, these facilities were more than adequate to serve all the children in the city who might benefit from its services. Initially, the special school facilities were intended to accommodate children with all degrees of severity of MR, but these plans were changed because of concerns about stigma. The planners decided that the special school would present a more favorable image in the community if children with more severe MR, whose appearance was more likely to be atypical, were placed in a Junior Occupation Center. The staff at the JOC were not teachers trained in special education, but child care workers who could attend to the special needs of children with severe MR.

Table 15.1 Paths through mental retardation (MR) services in childhood, characteristics of the children, and their family backgrounds

Type of service			Personal characteristics			
			Gender		IQ	
Initial placement		Final placement	M	F	Median	% <50
		Day				
1. Spec. school (n = 19)	→	Regular school	11	8	68	0
2. Spec. school (n = 140)	→	Spec. school	74	66	66	2
3. Spec. school (n = 15)	→	Jr. Occ. Center (JOC)	10	14	44	67
4. Jr. Occ. Center (n = 9)	↗					
		Residential				
5. Children's Inst. (n = 12)	→	Children's Inst.	11	3	39	100
6. Spec. school → JOC (n = 2)	↗					
7. Spec. school (n = 2)	→	Boarding JOC	3	1	40	100
8. Spec. school → JOC (n = 1)	↗					
9. JOC (n = 1)	↗					
10. Spec. school (n = 3)	→	Boarding spec. school	2	1	52	0
11. Spec. school (n = 6)	→	Adolescent Unit in adult institution	6	0	63	0
12. Spec. school (n = 2)	→	Remand home	1	1	67	0
13. Spec. school (n = 1)	→	Residence for people with epilepsy	0	1	67	0
		Home				
14. Home care (n = 7)	→	Home care	3	5	25	100
15. Spec. school → JOC (n = 1)	↗					

Both of these day service facilities were the general responsibility of the head of the special school, which ensured close communication and cooperation between them. It was an established policy that children be given the benefit of the doubt and, whenever possible, be placed initially at the special school. Because of concerns about stigma and the public image of the special school, some children, whose appearance resembled the general stereotype of mental retardation, were placed directly into the JOC without an initial trial at the special school. According to a second policy, evaluation of each

Table 15.1 (continued)

Childhood behavior disturbance		Childhood epilepsy	Cerebral palsy	Speech/ no speech	Down syndrome	Family stability		Deaths
Median	% Mod.-Sev.	% Mod.-Sev.	% Mod.-Sev.	%	*N*	Median	% 3–5	*N*
1	31	5	0	0	0	2.5	50	0
1	31	7	6	0	0	2	42	0
1	27	4	8	5	7	1	27	1
5	80	100	36	50	3	1.5	30	2
3	50	0	0	0	0	5	75	0
3	100	0	0	0	0	3	67	0
5	100	33	17	0	0	3	67	0
5	100	0	0	0	0	4	100	0
3	100	100	0	0	0	4	100	0
0	0	75	63	75	1	1	0	3

child's functioning would continue after the initial placement, that is, throughout childhood. We will see how well these policies worked later in the chapter.

In addition to learning school subjects, these children also needed social training. The children at the special school were taken on educational excursions, involved in sports activities with other schools, and taken camping during the summer holidays. Because of their many social problems (see Chapter 14), three full-time social workers were assigned to get to know them and provide assistance when needed, including helping the young people in the transition from childhood into adulthood.

Residential services. Some children with MR were excluded from the educational system, either because they were too limited to benefit from it or because the educational system was unable to cope with their severe behavior disturbance and epilepsy. For these children, the only services available were residential, and they were of several kinds. One institution, for children with severe disabilities, emphasized custodial and physical care. A residential JOC run by a voluntary agency provided care for other children. In addition, although it was intended mainly for adults with MR, there was a large regional institution that had an adolescent unit, and some older children were sent there. Outside Aberdeen, regional boarding schools provided care to children with mild MR who lived in areas lacking a local special school. For various reasons, a few children from Aberdeen were sent to some of these schools. Two children from the special school were sent by the courts to remand homes for juvenile delinquents, and one child was placed in a residential facility that treated children and adults with epilepsy.

Care in parents' home. Some parents, whose only service option was to put their children into residential care, decided instead to look after them at home, without help from the services described above. This situation changed during the years those in the study population were children. A voluntary organization established a day center for the care of children with severe disabilities, enabling parents who gave their children continuous care at home to have some respite for two half-days a week. The agency demonstrated that there was a need for this form of care, and city authorities later established a five-day-a-week day care facility for children with severe disabilities.

Personal Characteristics of the Children

We selected seven particular characteristics for analysis because we felt that they might influence the paths children followed through MR services.

Gender. For each path, we provide sex distributions.

IQ. For those in each path, we show the median childhood IQ and the percentage with IQ's below 50 (severe mental retardation).

Behavior disturbance. We used the 6-point scale of severity of overall behavior disturbance, described in Chapter 8, which ranged from 0 (no evidence of disturbance) to 5 (severe behavior disturbance). The median score and the percentage with scores of 3 or more (moderate to severe) are shown in the table.

Epilepsy. We used the 4-point scale of disability due to epilepsy described in Chapter 9, which ranged from 0 (none) to 3 (severe). We show the percentage with moderate-to-severe disability due to epilepsy.

Cerebral palsy (CP). We assessed CP according to degree of functional disability using a 4-point scale ranging from 0 (no CP) to 3 (severe disability). The percentage with moderate-to-severe disability due to CP is shown.

No speech. An assessment of verbal communication was carried out for the study subjects at age 22 (see Chapter 10). We inferred that those who had no speech at 22 also had no speech as children, and in some cases, this was confirmed from records. We show the percentage with no speech in each path.

Down syndrome. For each path we indicate the number of children with Down syndrome.

Mortality

In each path, we note the number of children who died.

Family Upbringing

To provide a summary indicator of each individual's upbringing, we used the measure of Family Stability described in Chapter 14. This was rated on a 5-point scale from 1 (stable) to 5 (markedly unstable). The median rating and the percentage with a rating of 3 to 5 on the scale is shown.

Most of the children whose first MR placement was the special school had previously attended regular classes. They were transferred to the special school only after it was clear that they were unable to cope and had been given a full evaluation, including psychometric testing. In some cases, children remained in regular classes for several years before their MR became clear. In others, MR was recognized early, but the child was placed in a regular class in line with the "benefit of the doubt" policy of the education authorities. Placements at the JOC tended to be early in the school years, and some placements into institutions occurred before school entry age.

Paths through Children's Mental Retardation Services

When we have briefly outlined the various paths through children's services and the numbers of children in these paths, we will discuss them in more detail. We will also examine the children's histories to see how these influenced the paths into which the children were placed.

The first of these final placements (Table 15.1, lines 1–3) show the various paths of children who were in day services only. By far the largest number of children with MR (n = 140) were placed in the special school initially and remained there until school-leaving age (line 2). Nineteen children at the special school improved sufficiently in their class work to be transferred back to regular classes (line 1). Fifteen were unable to cope with the program at the special school and were transferred to the JOC. The only other children who remained in day services throughout were the 9 who were placed in the JOC initially and remained there until school-leaving age (line 4). In all, 183 children (83 percent) spent all their school-age years in day services.

A childhood spent exclusively in residential care was uncommon; only 12 children (5 percent) had this experience (line 5). Lines 6 to 13 show a variety of paths in which children received both day and residential services (n = 18, 8 percent). Lines 14 and 15 represent paths in which children were wholly or primarily cared for in their parents' homes (n = 8, 4 percent).

These paths demonstrate the importance of the special school—in all, 192 children (87 percent) spent some time there—and that continuing evaluation of each child's functioning after initial placement in MR services was carried out.

Personal Characteristics of Children in the Various Paths

Children who stayed in day services (lines 1–4). The personal characteristics and family stability of the children whose final placement was the special school and those who returned to regular schools were remarkably similar, providing few clues about why children followed one path or the other. Both had IQ's at the upper end of the mild MR range, little behavior disturbance, and similar scores on family stability. One difference was the absence of cerebral palsy among those who returned to regular schools.

Included among the children whose final placement was the JOC, as would be expected, were many more with severe MR than among those in the other two day-service paths. Their other personal characteristics were similar to those whose final placement was the special school, with the exception of Down syndrome. This difference may have been due in part to the educational authorities' practice of keeping children who bore the clear stigmata of mental retardation out of the special school, in order to gain acceptance by teachers in regular schools and by the general public. While a final placement in the JOC may have been appropriate for children with Down syndrome, it is significant that none were given the "benefit of the doubt" and placed, at least initially, in the special school. After the conclusion of our follow-up study, the parents of a child with Down syndrome successfully challenged this exclusionary practice, but the special school had by that time won a large measure of acceptance in the community.

The decision to keep children at the special school, return them to a regular school, or transfer them to the JOC appeared to rest mainly on ongoing evaluation of each child's performance. The decisions were made by the principal, in consultation with teachers, the school psychologist, the school medical officer, and the parents. The low rate of behavior disturbance was explained by the fact that children with whom the day services could not cope were removed. The wide range on the family stability measure suggests that families were not a factor in placement. For various reasons, some of the children who attended day services were unable to live with parents, and they resided in various small hostels run by the local government or private agencies and intended for all children in need of substitute homes, whether they had mental retardation or not.

Final Placement in Residential Services (Lines 5–13)

The Children's Institution (lines 5 and 6). For twelve children, the institution was their only placement. The remaining two children, with prior placement in day services, had histories of deteriorating functioning. All twelve had severe MR, and they had more disabilities than children in any other final placement except those cared for at home. For most, it was the characteristics of the child that precipitated the placement and not instability in the family.

The median age at which children were placed in the institution was 5 years, and ranged from eighteen months to 9 years, a younger entry age than any other form of service. The two youngest placements had been abandoned, and both children showed clear evidence of disability.

Severe behavior problems were major factors in the institutional placement of six children, which added to their burden of care resulting from their other disabilities. One child had severe epilepsy, was incontinent during seizures, and smeared his feces wherever he could reach. His mother was gradually worn down by the stress, and on the advice of the family doctor, the parents agreed to place him in the institution at age 6. Another child, who exhibited highly aggressive and destructive behavior, had cerebral palsy. The family coped as long as they were able to but finally agreed to place their child in the institution at age 5. A third child screamed almost constantly. It was more than the father could stand, and against the wishes of his wife, he instigated residential placement, and the mother finally acquiesced. More than one mother said that institutional placement was the only recourse, because the demands of caring for her child were so overwhelming that she neglected the rest of the family.

With one exception, all the children placed in the institution had clear, visible stigmata associated with MR. Given the contemporary view of MR and a pessimistic prognosis, these stigmata may have contributed to the placement decisions.

Because mental retardation is the focus of the present study, it is natural to attribute a central causal role in institutional placement to the child with MR and to neglect other forms of stress experienced by the families. But this was not always the case. For example, one mother was also caring for her own father, who lived with the family, was largely bedridden, and needed nursing care.

Boarding Junior Occupation Center (lines 7–9). The few children placed at the Boarding JOC entered at an older age than the children placed in the institution. The median age was 13, with a range from 7 to 14 years. All had earlier placements in day services and all had severe MR, but except for the 50 percent who had behavior disturbance, they had no other disabilities. The rate of unstable families was high. Three of the children had been living with family substitutes, who were unable to continue providing care. The fourth was placed because his father's work took the family to various parts of the world and the frequent moves were very disruptive for the child.

Special boarding school (line 10). The three children who were placed at the special boarding school went there late in their school careers. The median age was 14 and the range from 10 to 16 years. All three had IQ's at the lower end of the mild MR range, and all had moderate-to-severe behavior disturbance but no other disability. In two cases, the teachers in the special school were unable to cope with the behavior of the children, and the transfer was initiated by the education authorities. In the third case, the family had experienced a series of catastrophes with their other children, and the mother had mental health problems.

Adolescent unit at the adult institution (line 11). The six children who were placed in the adolescent unit of the adult institution were all boys, and all had previously been at the special school. Apart from one boy with epilepsy and cerebral palsy, the only other disability was behavior disturbance, which was found in three of the boys. One constantly ran away from the substitute home where he had been living and refused to attend school, and another had problems with unacceptable sexual behavior. Still another boy concealed and did not take prescribed medication, and this led to the onset of severe epileptic attacks. These children were older, ranging in age from 12 to 16, with a median age of 13.5 years.

Homes for delinquent children (line 12). Two children were committed to a remand home for juvenile delinquents by the courts. Both came from unstable families, and both were age 13 on entry.

Residence for individuals with epilepsy (line 13). One girl who had epilepsy came from a family that was encountering many problems. When her behavior became too difficult for teachers at the special school to handle, the education authorities and her parents agreed that she should be placed outside the family home. At age 14, she was sent to a residence for children and adults with epilepsy.

We have gone into considerable detail in describing various residential placements in order to illustrate the heterogeneity of the children in residential care and their families. In eighteen of the thirty cases, the transfers originated from the special school because of behavior problems they could not deal with. The forms of services and the ways in which they are organized will vary by time and place. It is likely, however, that the diverse needs and problems of the children will remain relatively constant.

Children cared for at home (lines 14 and 15). The eight children who were cared for at home had high mortality rates, but in some respects, they were similar to those placed in the children's institution. Both sets of children had severe and multiple disabilities; the one difference was the absence of behavior disturbance among the children cared for at home. Both sets of children had been excluded from the special educational system, which left parents with only two choices—to place their child in an institution or care for them at home. Accounts from parents who kept their children at home make clear the high physical and psychological cost of doing so, and it increased as the children grew older and larger. Some families came close to breakdown, because the children needed almost constant care, which prevented any kind of social life or pursuit of personal interests, and rendered normal household and shopping activities very difficult. Some parents reported that loss of sleep added to their stress. Often relatives, friends, and neighbors provided help and respite, and some home help was provided by the local government. The eventual establishment of child care for two half-days a week by a voluntary agency was helpful, and some parents placed their children in the institution for a week or two in order to get some relief.

Heroic efforts were needed on the part of the parents, especially the mothers, to care for their children at home. After the follow-up study was completed, the local government took over responsibility for day care of children with severe and multiple disabilities who did not have behavior problems. We were told a story that illustrates the close cooperation among the city agencies. The Lord Mayor had a very large and expensive car that was used only on ceremonial occasions. When he learned of the establishment of the day facility for children with severe disabilities and the shortage of vehicles for transporting them back and forth, he arranged to have his car used for this purpose.

Personal Characteristics That May Have Influenced Placements

IQ. Of the thirty children whose final placement was in residential care, eighteen had severe MR; fourteen of them were placed in the children's institution, and the remaining four were sent to the boarding JOC. The twelve children with mild MR were distributed among four different kinds of residences. Residential care in childhood, then, was by no means only for children with severe MR.

Gender. For the total population of children with MR in the study, the ratio of boys to girls was 1.2 to 1.0. This ratio varied according to type of path through services. For those in all forms of residential care, males, with a ratio of 3.3 to 1.0, were overrepresented. Among children at the JOC or cared for at home, females were overrepresented, with ratios of girls to boys of 1.4 to 1.0 and 1.7 to 1.0, respectively. For the children whose final placement was a regular school or the special school, the ratios of boys to girls were 1.4 to 1.0 and 1.1 to 1.0, respectively.

Behavior. Children in all forms of residential care had higher rates of behavior disturbance than children in day services or cared for at home.

Down syndrome. The highest concentration of children with Down syndrome was at the Junior Occupation Center (seven of eleven). There were only two other paths in which children with Down syndrome were found: three were in the institution throughout, since infancy, and one was cared for at home.

Mortality. Six children died. The highest mortality rate was among the children cared for at home (three of eight). The next highest rate was at the children's institution, where two of fourteen died. The remaining death was that of a child at the JOC.

Adult Histories in Mental Retardation Services

The Social Context

Day services. Two Senior Occupation Centers (SOC's) provided services five days a week during normal working hours. Built to accommodate adults with different degrees of mobility, they first opened a few years before the oldest members of the study population reached school-leaving age (15–16). Most of the young adults who went to an SOC gained admittance as soon as they left children's day services. A few of the older study subjects experienced some delay before a place became available.

The stated aim of the SOC's was to enable all clients to find a place in society in which they would enjoy a measure of independence commensurate with their ability. Their programs emphasized the development of the social skills necessary for living in the community, including domestic and interpersonal skills, learning to use public transportation and function as a pedestrian, and learning various leisure activities. Trained teachers were not used, and no staff training courses were available at the time. Staff were chosen for their personal abilities, and training was informal and on-the-job. An additional and important function of the SOC's was to provide respite from care to parents.

It was soon clear that no single program would effectively meet the entire range of client needs. At one of the centers a special wing was added to provide for the needs of adults with the most serious and multiple disabilities, many of whom required close, continuous supervision and nursing care. Initially, also, the SOC's were not providing the kinds of training that more able young people needed to function in the community without MR services. A third SOC, developed to provide this sort of training, was opened shortly before the youngest adults in the study reached age 22.

Residential services. The main facility for residential care of adults with MR was a large, long-established regional institution under medical direction, located some distance from Aberdeen. The institution contained a unit for adolescents, as we noted in our description of children's services.

Eventually, some smaller residences for adults with MR were established within the city's boundaries. This was done as part of a continuing effort to move people from the regional institution back into the community and to assist some of them in managing without further services. The smaller community residences reflected an early stage in the movement away from the traditional large institutions.

A few places were available on training farms, run by voluntary agencies, to provide a sheltered environment for young men and training in farm work and horticulture commensurate with their abilities. To be accepted, they had to be physically able and exhibit good social behavior.

For all individuals with any history of adult MR services, we examined the amount of time they had spent in services. As we discovered, it was almost always either less than one third of the period from 15–16 to age 22 or more than two thirds. We refer to these as either short- or long-term services.

Short- and long-term services. There is an important difference between short-term placements in day services and those in residential services. In day services, the young adults and their parents were free to decide whether they stayed or left. In residential services, with the exception of the training farms, the length of stay was decided by the authorities in charge of the services and occasionally by the courts.

No adult MR services. As we have shown, approximately half of all the children placed in MR services did not continue on into adult services. In subsequent chapters we will examine what happened to them and to those who received only short-term adult services.

The adult service paths fall into five categories: short- and long-term day services, short- and long-term residential services, and no services. A few adults received both day and residential services. For ease of analysis, we assigned them to the service path in which they spent most of their time. Two women at the SOC, for example, were sent to the regional institution for a few months because of acute psychiatric problems.

Table 15.2 shows the individual paths from final MR service placements in childhood to placement in adult services or no services. Adult services are subdivided by whether they were day or residential and short- or long-term. Six children died, leaving a total of 215

Table 15.2 Paths from final placements in childhood to adult MR services and no services

Final childhood placements	Adult MR services: Day		Adult MR services: Residential		No services	Total
	Short-term	Long-term	Short-term	Long-term		
Returned to regular school	0	0	0	1	18	19
Special School or JOC	13	38	5	6	101	163
Residential	1	3	1	20	3	28
Home care	0	5	0	0	0	5
Total	14	46	6	27	122	215
Deaths in childhood						6
Total population						221

young people with histories of childhood MR who survived to age 16. Of the survivors, 43 percent were in some adult service. Almost twice as many were in day services than in residential services, and long-term three times more often than short-term. Adults in day services generally also had childhood histories of day services (81 percent), and adults in residential services largely had childhood histories of residential services (84 percent). Of the 57 percent of the young adults who received no adult services, 98 percent had a history of day services in childhood.

The surviving children cared for at home were all in long-term day care at a Senior Occupation Center as young adults, where, as we have noted, a special wing was set aside for those with severe and multiple disabilities.

Table 15.3 provides a more detailed picture of the paths through MR services from the final childhood placement to adult MR services and includes the same personal characteristics categories that were used to describe the children.

Personal Characteristics and Family Background

Between the ages of 15–16 and 22 years, the categories of gender, cerebral palsy, Down syndrome, and family upbringing did not change. Because no IQ's were obtained after age 15, we used childhood IQ. For the young adult period we obtained separate measures of behavior disturbance and disability due to epilepsy, and used these to cover the age range of 16–22. At age 22, an assessment of verbal communication was obtained (see Chapter 10 for a full description of the measure). Table 15.3 shows percentages for moderate-to-severe verbal communication disorders and notes the number of deaths and the paths in which they took place.

Adult MR Services and Factors That Influenced Placements

Day services, short-term. Some of the young adults who had short-term day placements entered the SOC several years after leaving school, following unsuccessful job careers. Others entered directly from school and then left for a variety of reasons: a few found jobs with the help of the day center staff or the social work department, and others left because they were discontented with SOC programs. In some cases, the parents considered the program inappropriate and encouraged their children to leave, or they themselves initiated the withdrawal. We noted earlier that males, all of whom had mild MR, predominated in short-term care. The programs at the SOC's, however, were oriented more to the interests of women and the needs of those with severe MR, and this may have accounted for the short stays of some of the men, especially those with higher IQ's.

Day services, long-term. For most of the young adults with severe MR, the local authorities and the parents agreed that placement in a Senior Occupation Center, without giving them a trial in the open job market, was in their best interests. These decisions were often based on the severity and sometimes multiplicity of disabilities. In contrast, some of the young people with mild MR had first attempted unsuccessfully to get or hold a job.

Residential services. For most of the young people who went from the children's institution to adult residences, the reasons for their childhood placements held when they became young adults: generally they required a level of care beyond the capacity of many families or there was no one to care for them because of family breakup or abandonment. In a few cases, the reasons were less apparent, and the history of childhood residential placement itself, combined with lack of an alternative, appeared to have contributed to the continuity of the placement.For some, mainly those with mild MR, the length of stay in adult residences was determined by the officials in charge, based on their judgment of whether the young adult gave evidence of being able to function in the community.

Twelve people in the adult institution had been in day services as children. These young adults had unstable family backgrounds and a high frequency of behavior disturbance. Six were placed as the result of a court order, five were committed by psychiatrists, and one had nowhere else to go because of family instability.

The role of the courts in placing young adults in MR institutions is a difficult one and may be illustrated by the Aberdeen experience. The courts required that the social work department furnish them with a history of each young adult who appeared before them who had earlier received services for children with MR. Judges had discretion to send these individuals to the MR institution or give them a sentence equivalent to that of someone with no history of MR. In some cases, the young adult was sentenced to the MR institution only

Table 15.3 Adult mental retardation services extended from final childhood placements, and the personal characteristics of the young adults ages 16–22 and their family backgrounds

		Personal characteristics			
		Gender		Childhood IQ	
Final childhood placement	Adult services	M	F	Median	% <50
Regular school	None	11	7	68	0
	Residential, long-term	0	1	68	0
Special day school	None	53	46	67	0
	Day, short-term	10	3	63	0
	Day, long-term	6	13	59	16
	Residential, short-term	2	1	71	0
	Residential, long-term	3	3	64.5	0
Jr. Occupation Center (JOC)	None	2	0	46	50
	Day long-term	6	13	40	79
	Residential, short-term	2	0	53.5	0
Institution	Residential, long-term	10	2	40	100
Boarding JOC	Day, long-term	0	1	40	100
	Residential, long-term	3	0	40	100
Boarding special school	Day, short-term	0	1	69	0
	Day, long-term	1	0	51	0
	Residential, long-term	1	0	52	0
Adolescent unit at adult institution	None	1	0	66	0
	Residential, short-term	1	0	67	0
	Residential, long-term	4	0	59	0
Remand home	None	1	1	67	0
Residence for epileptics	Day, long-term	0	1	67	0
Home care	Day, long-term	2	3	30	100

after repeated offenses. Of the seventeen who were sentenced to some kind of confinement by the courts, six were sent to the adult MR institution and eleven to young offenders institutions or prison. In the follow-up study population, judges sent young adult offenders with a history of mental retardation to the adult MR institution in only one third of their judgments.

The decision to place four of the young adults in the institution was made by doctors, social workers, and parents. In three of these

Table 15.3 (continued)

Personal characteristics									
Behavior disturbance age 16–22		Epilepsy age 16–22	Cerebral palsy	Verbal communi-cation disorder	Down syndrome	Family stability		Deaths
Median	% Mod./ Sev.	% Mod./ Sev.	% Mod./ Sev.	% Mod./ Sev.	*N*	Median	% 3–5	*N*
1	27	0	0	0	0	2	47	0
5	100	0	0	0	0	5	100	0
1	29	4	3	4	0	2	43	1
3	54	15	8	0	0	2	38	0
0	16	16	32	10	0	2	11	0
5	100	0	0	0	0	4	100	0
5	100	0	0	17	0	3	100	1
2	0	0	0	0	1	4	100	0
1	42	11	5	48	5	1	16	0
3	50	0	0	0	0	4	100	0
2	40	25	33	100	3	1.5	30	1
3	100	0	0	0	0	5	100	0
0	33	33	0	6	0	5	67	0
3	100	0	0	0	0	4	100	0
1	0	0	0	0	0	2	0	0
5	100	0	0	100	0	3	100	0
5	100	0	0	0	0	5	100	0
5	100	0	0	0	0	3	100	0
5	100	50	25	25	0	2.5	50	0
2.5	50	0	0	0	0	4	100	0
2	0	100	0	0	0	4	100	0
.5	25	100	100	80	1	1	0	1

cases, a contributing factor was fear that the continued behavior would lead to arrest and legal action. The main reason for placement of the remaining young adult in the institution was an unstable family. He had held a job for some time after leaving school, but then, unable to cope with the job, remained at home during the day with his mother and stepfather. When his mother died, his stepfather remarried, having agreed with the new wife that the stepson would be sent elsewhere. For lack of any other option, the stepson was taken into the adult institution until a more appropriate placement could be found for him.

Deaths. There were four deaths between the ages of 16 and 22 in the study population. Two were males with mild MR who had attended the special school: one was a known suicide, and the other a suspected suicide. The remaining deaths were of young adults with severe MR and multiple disabilities; one had been in an institution since childhood, and the other had been cared for at home during childhood and was in adult day care.

Characteristics of Those in Various Adult Paths

Severity of mental retardation. With one exception, everyone with severe MR went into long-term adult services. The exception was a young man with Down syndrome who helped out in a shop run by his parents. Of the rest, more went into day services ($n = 24$) than residential services ($n = 15$).

In long-term services, 54 percent of those in day care and 44 percent of those in residential care had mild MR; approximately half, that is, of those in long-term services had mild MR, a proportion that was larger than we had anticipated.

Gender. Because for a large majority, adult placements were of the same type as childhood placements, we again find that there were more males (79 percent) than females (40 percent) in adult residential care, and more females (60 percent) than males (21 percent) in adult day care. The majority of females in day care was entirely due to those in long-term services, where 69 percent were female. In short-term day services the males were in the majority with 71 percent. It was only in long-term day care that the majority were females.

Behavior. Because there was continuity in type of care between child and adult services, those in residential care showed more behavior disturbance than those in day care, even taking into account some changes in behavior disturbance between the two age periods. Twelve individuals who were in children's day services then went into adult residential services. They had higher rates of behavior disturbance than those who went into day service or no services.

Summary and Conclusions

Two primary factors, behavior disturbance and family instability, influenced whether children and young adults were placed in day services or residential services. During the school years, the behavior disturbance of some children was sufficiently severe that teachers were unable to cope with them, and they were transferred to a number of different residences. In many cases, the behavior disturbance also caused severe problems for parents. Most of the children with severe MR, even those with additional disabilities, were cared for in day facilities, while a few remained at home. What made it possible for parents and day services to cope with these children was the absence of behavior that created management problems.

Behavior was also an important factor in placement in adult residential services. As we have noted, in general, children in day and residential services continued in the same kind of adult service; for many also, there was continuity in their behavior disturbance from childhood to adulthood. The exceptions were the young people who were in day services in childhood, but were placed in residential services as young adults because of behavior disturbance.

Males were overrepresented in residential services and females in day services. In Chapter 8 we showed that there was no significant gender difference in the amount of overall behavioral disturbance. When we examined the type of disturbance, however, males had higher rates of antisocial behavior, and females higher rates of emotional disorders. Further, males with IQ's of 70 and above had more antisocial behavior than those with IQ's of less than 60. In the study population, twice as many males as females had IQ's of 70 and above. Gender differences in the manifestation of behavior disturbance, and the high ratio of males to females with IQ's of 70 and above help to explain the gender difference in residential and day care.

Apart from the children's institution, where entry was generally at an early age, placement of children in other kinds of residences occurred closer to the end of their schooling, when their added size and strength made management more difficult for their predominantly female caretakers. This occurred more frequently for males.

The disposition of cases of young people with MR who came before the courts illustrates the very difficult decisions confronting judges. In Aberdeen, when a person with a history of mental retardation was to appear before the court, the social work department was required to provide the judge with a history and evaluation of the young person. Without this information, judges would have been severely hampered in making their decisions and more likely to imprison young adults with MR, when such placements were inappropriate.

Family instability also played a role in residential placement. For the children placed in residential care in the preschool years, either behavior disturbance was not present or it was inadequate to explain the placement. Placement was apparently related to the clear, visible stigmata of MR, combined with parental abandonment or refusal to keep the child, although this does not explain why those placed in the children's institution at preschool ages were predominantly male. Gender in some way appeared to contribute to placement decisions for very young children. For one of the adults, the stepfather refused to continue to care for him after his mother died, which led to residential placement.

The frequency of family instability as a contributing factor in residential placement should be related to family life in the community. The families of the comparison population were generally stable and often included extended family relationships within the community. To the extent that there is less family stability in communities today than in Aberdeen at the time of the study, the need for some form of residential care for children and young adults with MR will be greater. If MR services are inadequate, generic services for children and young adults—for example, residences for juvenile delinquents and prisons—will of necessity have to include more individuals with mental retardation among their residents.

In view of the diverse characteristics of those they served, the experience of the Senior Occupation Centers clearly demonstrated that a single program was inadequate. The initial program focused mainly on social training and recreation. The first addition to this program was a special wing for the adults with severe multiple disabilities who needed nursing care and close supervision. The second was the opening of a new center that emphasized training for jobs and independent living. As the experience in Aberdeen suggests, adult day services must offer several different programs if they are to meet the range of needs among young adults.

The organization of MR services in any one time and place is largely determined by previous practices and available budgets. The major organizational changes appear to start with the recognition that something is very wrong with a particular service. But organized change is often difficult to achieve because vested interests will oppose it. An important factor in precipitating change is a powerful theoretical concept that is both appealing and readily grasped. Examples from the later part of this century in education are "normalization," "stigma," and "mainstreaming." The benefits of these and other concepts in helping to change the organization of MR services are real and important; their application, however, has had unintended consequences. A service created in response to a concept is often regarded as good and the previous service as bad; evidence showing the effectiveness of the new service and the faults of the previous service is sought through research. The concepts of normalization, stigma, and mainstreaming, for example, influenced the shift away from segregated arrangements for children with MR and toward their placement in regular classes. Only later was it recognized that children mainstreamed in regular classes were stigmatized because their more able classmates were aware of their lack of scholastic ability and social skills. Although particular concepts may seem to be panaceas to right wrongs, for those to whom the concept applies, the practical application may be harmful.

16

Job Histories

For men, jobs form the central role of adult life, defining not only economic but also social status. In Aberdeen at the time of the study, it was the community's expectation that when a couple married, and especially after they began to have children, the husband would be the primary breadwinner, and family status would derive largely from his job. For women, the job role was perceived differently. While they were single, and after marriage while they still had no children, young women expected to work, and the kinds of jobs they held were important economically and socially. After marriage and children, however, they generally left the labor force and did not work outside the home, at least until their children were in school. Because most young women expected to marry and have children, they envisioned their future job careers in shorter perspective. The children of the women in the follow-up study were mainly infants.

For adults who had been judged to have mild mental retardation (MR) during childhood, an important determinant of their need for adult MR services was whether, after leaving school, they would be able to obtain and hold a job. For those who did, the kinds of jobs they obtained, how long they held them, and how much time they spent unemployed influenced the degree to which they became independent.

Young people with MR may have problems as they enter the work force. The intellectual and scholastic incompetence that caused them to be identified as MR during their school years is likely to continue to cause difficulty for them in jobs that require literacy, numerical skills, and facility with language.

One consequence of the industrial revolution was the development of "scientific management." Jobs were analyzed and reconstituted so that workers needed only minimal skills and thus less job training time. According to Littler and Saloman (1985), this provided the rationale for the assembly line organization of jobs in discrete steps that did not generally require intellectual and scholastic competence. Rosenbrock (1985) suggested that many assembly line jobs might be more suited to people with MR: "slight mental retardation . . . often enables a person to do tedious work which would handicap a 'normal' worker because of the monotony" (p. 163).

The concept of "incompetence" focuses on the individual, whereas the changes stemming from "scientific management" include general, individual, and social factors, such as the physical conditions of the environment (heat, light and air quality), the physical demands made on the employee, and the spacial and social relationships among workers and between workers and equipment. We took these factors into account in studying the job histories of young persons with MR in the years after leaving the special school.

The Present Study

Of those with job histories of any kind, the large majority received no mental retardation services after leaving school. These individuals, who will be the primary focus of this chapter, were the adults to whom Gruenberg (1964) referred when he questioned whether or not they were still handicapped. To determine the similarities and differences in the job histories of those with and without mild mental retardation, we will include the comparison subjects. For the small minority who had some jobs but also received adult MR services, we will briefly describe only their histories and not whether they differed from comparisons.

To provide an adequate picture of job histories, it was important to examine subjective measures of how the young people felt about their job histories, and how they evaluated them, as well as more objective measures, such as how long they worked. Because the job histories covered a seven-year period, it was also important to include some measures, such as amount of time employed and unemployed, that spanned individual job careers. These measures, however, do not provide information on the kinds of work the young people were doing at age 22. It has been suggested that because young people with MR learn at a slower rate than peers who do not have MR, it takes them longer to adapt to the standards required for adequate functioning in a job. At the time of the study, school-leaving age in Aberdeen was 15 or 16 for all the children with histories of mental retardation. The transition from the world of school to the world of work may have been more difficult at that age than at an older school-leaving age. Job performance at age 22 may therefore provide a better indication of what the young people were capable of doing, so we will also examine jobs at this age.

Young People with Mental Retardation

With one exception, no one with severe MR had any job history. Among those with mild MR, the results deal with 89 males and 65 females who survived until age 22. They were subdivided into those who received no MR services after leaving school, those who had some job histories but also spent some time in adult services, and those who had no job histories and were in adult services throughout the postschool period. The numbers and percentages of males and females in these three categories are shown in Table 16.1. More females than males had no job histories.

Nonretarded Comparisons

In Aberdeen as in the entire United Kingdom at this time, students in their last year of regular secondary school took national exami-

Table 16.1 Job and service histories of adults with mental retardation by gender (percentages in parentheses)

	Males	Females
Received no adult MR services (have job histories)	60 (67)	40 (62)
Some adult MR services and some job history	14 (16)	5 (8)
Adult MR services predominantly	15 (17)	20 (30)
Total	89	65

nations. If passed, they awarded two levels of qualifications, which were prerequisites for entry into further education and training and into certain skilled jobs. None of the young people with mental retardation had achieved these educational qualifications. It is reasonable to expect that young adults who do leave school with these qualifications will have jobs with higher levels of skill at age 22 than the young people with MR. For this reason, we restricted the comparisons to those who left school without qualifications (33 males and 19 females), but because of this selection we lost case-by-case matching on year of birth and social class. We therefore examined whether either of these variables had different distributions in the young people with MR and the remaining comparisons, and whether either variable was related to any of the job history variables. None of these analyses yielded significant results, suggesting that relinquishing matching on year of birth and social class did not bias our findings.

Measures of Job Histories

We developed measures to examine the following questions:

1. How much of the individual's time between leaving school and age 22 was spent employed, unemployed, or out of the labor force?
2. What kinds of work did the individual perform in the jobs held?
3. How similar or different were the job histories of those with MR and the comparisons?

Objective Measures

Percentage of time employed. The number of months employed divided by the number of months between leaving school and 22 years, 3 months of age.

Percentage of time unemployed. The number of months out of work but seeking employment divided by months in the labor force (defined as time employed plus time unemployed). For those with no MR services, the percentage of time employed was generally the inverse of the percentage of time unemployed. For those who received MR services, however, this inverse relationship did not hold because of the time they spent out of the labor force and in adult services.

Percentage of time out of the work force. The number of months spent neither employed nor unemployed but seeking employment divided by the number of months between leaving school and 22 years, 3 months of age. We excluded time as a housewife and time in full-time education, because the former is alternative unpaid work and the latter contributed to more skilled job performance.

Job turnover. The number of jobs an individual held per year in the labor force.

Level of job skill. These included *skilled* work, which required some formal qualification obtained through training, including apprenticeships, evening classes, or work-release time for training (for example, butcher, printer, baker, electrician, shorthand typist, policeman); *semiskilled* work—manual jobs that involved the acquisition of skills directly related to the specific job and generally acquired through job experience (for example, machine operator, assistant cook, waiter or waitress, shop assistant, carpet fitter, van driver); and *unskilled* work, which required no skills or only those easily acquired in a short time. Jobs were manual, simple, and generally repetitive (for example, laborer, cleaner, and remover).

The level of job skill at age 22 gave a good picture of an individual's career course over the previous 6 to 7 years. With few exceptions, those in unskilled jobs had held unskilled jobs throughout, and those with semiskilled or skilled jobs started out in unskilled jobs.

Interpersonal skills. Each job was classified according to whether the work required interpersonal skills—such as dealing with customers or clients—beyond those generally needed in working alongside others and in relating to supervisors or employers (for example, receptionist, shop assistant, bus conductor, supervisor, waiter or waitress, sales representative, nurse's aide). Jobs not requiring interpersonal skills were those in which the work dealt primarily with objects (for example, cleaner, dishwasher, laborer).

Take-home pay. Based on information for the job an individual held at age 22. The period 1966 through 1977 was one of currency inflation, so take-home pay for those in the older and younger birth cohorts was not comparable. To take account of inflation, we therefore converted take-home pay to a standard score based on the means and standard deviations for each of the five birth cohorts by sex.

Part-time jobs. The number of part-time jobs an individual held in addition to full-time jobs.

Apprenticeships. Whether individuals entered and completed apprenticeships.

For all these measures, we determined whether there were group differences between those with MR and comparisons. This is how previous investigators have presented their results, and these are the kinds of data from which reviewers have drawn their conclusions; the reviewers' conclusions, however, were couched in terms of how many individuals with mental retardation had made a satisfactory adjustment as adults. To compare our results with their conclusions, we needed some way of determining, for each individual, whether he or she was functioning in ways that were similar to or deviant from their peers who did not have mental retardation.

Job history deviance. Determining individual deviance through measures of *unemployment, turnover,* and *time out of the labor force.* From a societal point of view of what constitutes a preferred labor force, it is reasonable to posit low rather than high unemployment, less turnover rather than more, and less time out of the labor force. By contrast, from a societal view of the needs of an industrial economy, all categories of level-of-job skill, take-home pay, and jobs that do and do not require interpersonal skills are needed.

To establish measures of individual deviance, we calculated percentile distributions of unemployment, turnover, and time out of the labor force for the nonretarded comparisons. We then defined deviance as beyond the ninetieth percentile for the distributions of the comparisons of each sex. This definition has four advantages. First, it describes conditions prevailing at the time and place of the study, thus providing a basis for comparing one community and time with another. Second, the conditions of the labor force are likely to differ along gender lines, and separate ratings of deviance may be determined for men and for women. Although direct comparisons between men and women are inappropriate, the deviance ratings provide a way of asking whether the frequency of deviance from the same sex norm is similar or different for men and women with mental retardation. Third, in addition to examining deviance on unemployment, job turnover, and time out of the labor force separately, we could study deviance across the three measures for each person. Fourth, deviance as we have defined it is not unique to people with mental retardation. The statistical procedures and testing of difference are described fully in Richardson, Koller, and Katz (1988). Here we will only state whether or not differences were found.

Kinds of Jobs. In reviewing the specific jobs held by the entire study population, we compiled lists of over nine hundred different jobs for males and over five hundred for females. From these lists, we developed a set of job classifications.

Laborers. Under supervision, laborers performed manual work requiring physical strength, such as lifting, carrying, digging, and stacking, frequently outdoors. They differed from porters, who often had some autonomy and carried out more specific tasks.

Delivery boys. These were entry-level jobs requiring no skills or experience. Delivery boys worked in vans or trucks bringing various types of goods to private homes or businesses under the direction of the van or truck driver.

Cleaners. In these jobs, the primary task was cleaning and removing garbage or trash from offices or homes.

Workers. These were jobs, such as "farm worker," that included the term in the title. The work, generally done in factories, on farms, or for small businesses, was not specialized, as in "division of labor" below, generally required little skill or experience, and was carried out under supervision.

Division of labor. In these jobs, production was broken down, as on an assembly line, into specific tasks in the manufacture of a product. The worker carried out one or more specific and often repetitive tasks. The jobs required varying degrees of skill and experience, for example, stapling boxes together, killing and gutting chickens, filleting fish, operating a machine, or sewing soles on slippers.

Porters. Porters moved things from one place to another. The settings, which varied widely, included railway stations, hotels, and factories.

Food and drink services. These jobs involved the preparation and serving of meals and drinks. Examples include waiters, stewards on ships, cooks, and bar staff.

Trainee/Learner. This category included people working under supervision, with informal training on the job as a component. This training differed from that in apprenticeships, where it led to formal qualifications.

Assistants. Assistants helped and were supervised by another worker. Although the job description included no explicit training component, the assistant may have learned something about the work. Examples include assistants to welders, electricians, agricultural workers, butchers, and machine repair personnel.

Apprentices. Under a formal agreement with an employer, apprentices worked under skilled craftsmen to learn the particular craft or trade. Apprenticeships lasted several years and involved classes at technical colleges. To complete their training, individuals had to pass examinations to show that they met local or national standards.

Armed Forces. These were jobs performed in the service of the army, navy, or air force.

Merchant Navy. These were jobs carried out on merchant ships.

Drivers. These workers drove lorries, trucks, tractors, and fork lifts. The job was limited mainly to driving.

Delivery workers. These workers were also drivers, but they drove vans (for the post office and for dairy and food companies, for example) that delivered goods and packages to private homes and businesses, often assisted by a delivery boy.

Sales. These jobs involved selling in shops and supermarkets, and over the telephone, and pumping petrol (gasoline) for cars at a service station.

Supervisors. Supervisors had primary responsibility for directing work done by others. Examples include managers, foremen, and charge hands.

Journeymen and artisans. These jobs, whose skills were manual, followed some form of training, often an apprenticeship, that required a certification process. They included butcher, carpenter, confectioner, and hairdresser.

Office workers. These jobs included any work in an office, other than manager and supervisor, such as typist, secretary, receptionist, dispatcher, ledger clerk.

Warehouse and storemen. People in these jobs were responsible for organizing and dispersing parts needed in factories and repair shops, and maintaining inventories of goods or parts.

Packers. These were jobs in which the work was exclusively packing food or industrial products.

Subjective Measures

Reasons for leaving jobs. The measure of job turnover provides information on the number of jobs individuals left but not on their reasons for leaving, which might include being fired for poor performance, leaving for a more attractive or higher paid job, or being laid off from a seasonal job. We wanted to know the reasons young people gave for leaving jobs and whether they would differ for those with mental retardation and for the comparisons. For each job they left, they were asked their reasons for leaving. (The question did not apply to those who remained in a single job.) The number of jobs young people left varied widely, so that those with a higher job turnover rate gave more reasons for leaving than those with a lower turnover rate. In addition, some gave single reasons and some gave multiple reasons for leaving a job. The average number given by those with MR and the comparisons, both male and female, was similar, so the two groups may be compared.

It is possible that one person might give the same reason for leaving several jobs, while another might give a particular reason only once or twice. When this happened, the occurrence of these reasons would be heavily influenced by that one individual. We examined the data to determine whether this happened.

Jobs liked most and least. By asking the young people in the study to choose the jobs they liked most and least, and why they made these choices, we hoped to learn about which aspects of jobs, both positive and negative, were important to them. Clearly, only those who had held several jobs could give meaningful responses.

To examine the reasons for leaving jobs and, separately, the reasons individuals gave for choosing particular jobs as most- and least-liked, several readers reviewed all responses and developed a set of categories. We looked closely at the reliability of the coding of responses into categories and found it to be satisfactory.

For both analyses, we used the total number of responses as the denominator, and the number in each category as the numerator, yielding the percentages of all responses in each category.

The Setting

Chapter 4 provides a general description of Aberdeen at the time of the study. The job histories of the study population must be seen in the context of the kinds of work available to young people in the late 1960s and early 1970s in Aberdeen. The absence of educational qualifications among the study population served to exclude them from many of the more skilled and higher-paying jobs. To put together a picture of the kinds of employment they were able to obtain, we compiled a list of all the employers who had hired study subjects, both those with MR and the comparisons. The following description is based on this employer list.

Aberdeen is a seaport on the east coast of Scotland. As we have mentioned, the port has been the basis for a variety of jobs related to catching and processing fish, general shipping, ship repairing and building, and oil production in the North Sea. The hinterland to the west of Aberdeen is an area of agriculture and forestry. Aberdeen, along with its environs, is home to a variety of industries, a seat of government, and a tourist center.

The production and processing of foods and beverages were major sources of employment. This industry, in fact, provided almost half of all employment for the study population under consideration here. In the food industry, the predominant job was fish processing, which provided more than twice as many jobs as any other form of employment. The nine largest sources of employment, ranked from most to least, were fish processing, wholesale and retail trade, manufacturing textiles and clothing, manufacturing paper products, the building trades, manufacturing and processing of beverages, sawmills and wood products, restaurants and other eating places, and the offshore oil industry. Males were more frequently employed in farming, fishing, meat processing, beverage manufacture and processing, the building trades, and heavy industry; females in fish processing, miscellaneous food processing, manufacture of paper products, wholesale and retail trades, restaurants and eating places, and hospitals.

Adults with Mental Retardation Who Received No Adult Services

Job histories. The interests of the community are best served by a low rate of unemployment, a generally low job turnover, and little time out of the labor force. We chose to examine these three aspects of job histories over the age span of 15 or 16 to 22, for both the young people with MR who received no adult MR services (hereafter called "no services") and the comparisons. Table 16.2 shows the amount of unemployment, job turnover, and time out of the job market. The only significant differences we found between the no services and the comparisons were more unemployment among the no-service males and more time out of the labor force among the no-service females.

Job deviance. In order to understand the estimates of deviance, it was first necessary to examine the conditions in the labor force at the time those in the study population worked, in the place they worked, and in the kinds of work they performed. The range and median of the rates on unemployment, turnover, and time out of the labor force for the comparisons shown in Table 16.2 provide an estimate of the conditions in which the no-service young people were likely to be employed. They show low rates of unemployment and little time out of the labor force. There is no basis for comparing these job turnover rates with those in other communities because such information is not published. As we explained earlier in discussing methods, the distributions of unemployment, turnover, and time out of the labor force for the comparisons provide the basis for our definition of deviance (that is, beyond the ninetieth percentile of the comparisons' distributions on the measures).

Among the no-service young people, 22 percent of the males and 18 percent of the females were deviant on unemployment (the ninetieth percentile for the comparison subjects on unemployment was 8.9 percent for males and 3.5 percent for females). On job turnover, 12 percent of the males and 10 percent of the females were deviant (the ninetieth percentile for the comparison subjects on time out was 12.4 percent for males and 2.3 percent for females). Across the three measures of deviance, 67 percent of the no-service males and 63 percent of the females were not deviant on any of the measures, and 7 percent of the males and 13 percent of the females were deviant on two or three of the measures.

Table 16.2 Unemployment, job turnover, and time out of the labor force for no services MR and comparisons, by gender

	Males				Females			
	No Services (n = 60)		Comparisons (n = 33)		No Services (n = 40)		Comparisons (n = 19)	
Job measure	Range	Median	Range	Median	Range	Median	Range	Median
Time unemployed	0–60%	1.3%	0–11%	0	0–16%	0	0–7%	0
Job turnover (No. jobs/yr.)	0–4.29	.59	.14–4.28	.439	0–12	.68	0–2.29	.48
Time out of labor force (%)[a]	0–43%	0	0–25%	0	0–99%	0	0–3%	0

a. Excluding time spent as housewife or in further education.

For the measures that follow, there is no societal expectation that everyone acts in the same way. Rather, to have an effective work force, a diversity of job roles is necessary, so a deviance score in not meaningful.

Interpersonal skills. Some jobs require interpersonal skills in carrying out their activities. Because mental retardation can affect social competence, we expected that it would be more difficult for young adults with MR to obtain and hold jobs involving interpersonal skills. Our expectation was confirmed for both males and females. The no-service group held jobs requiring interpersonal skills significantly less often than the comparisons. More than 80 percent of this group had never had jobs requiring interpersonal skills, with no significant gender difference. Among the comparisons, significantly fewer of the males (33 percent) than females (76 percent) held jobs requiring interpersonal skills.

Part-time and full-time jobs. Among males, some history of part-time work in addition to a full-time job was found significantly more often for the comparisons (42 percent) than for the no-service group (15 percent). For females, there was no significant difference.

Kinds of Job Held. Table 16.3 shows the percentages, by gender, of kinds of jobs held by the no-service group and the comparison group. The denominator is the total number of jobs held by each group. As might be expected, there were considerable gender differences. The only kind of job held with any frequency by all groups (males and females, no-service and comparison) was "division of labor" employment. In general, for both sexes, jobs requiring more skills were more often held by the comparisons. Among the males, the comparisons held jobs as supervisors, journeymen and artisans, warehouse and storemen, apprentices, and salesmen more often than the no-service group, who more often worked as laborers, cleaners, and workers.

Among the females, the comparisons more frequently had jobs in sales (26 percent) and office work (18 percent). Less than 1 percent of the no-service females held either of these kinds of jobs. They tended to work in cleaning, packing, and division of labor jobs.

Apprenticeships. Apprenticeships provided the path to many skilled jobs, but only if they were completed successfully. Table 16.3 shows the percentage of those who were apprentices, although it does not show how many completed their apprenticeship. Among no-

Table 16.3 Kinds of jobs held by those with MR who disappeared from services and comparisons, by gender (rounded to nearest percent)

	Males		Females	
Job	No Service (n = 60)	Comparisons (n = 40)	No Service (n = 40)	Comparisons (n = 19)
Message boys	7	6		
Delivery boys	2	3		
Laborers	19	7		
Cleaners	5	1	7	
Workers	15	9	10	8
Division of Labor	22	17	43	15
Porters	3	2		
Food and drink services	3	2	6	5
Packers	0	0	27	10
Trainee/Learner	4	2	1	5
Assistant	6	4		
Armed forces	1	3		
Merchant Navy	<1	2		
Delivery	3	3		3
Drivers	3	5		
Sales	1	7	1	26
Apprentices (see text)	5	18	0	5
Warehouse and Storemen	2	5	1	
Journeymen and Artisans	0	3		5
Office workers	0	0	1	18
Supervisors	<1	3	0	0
Other	2	2	2	
Number of jobs	189	83	125	39

service males, none of the 17 percent who entered apprenticeships completed them. Among the comparisons, of the 45 percent who entered apprenticeships, 18 percent completed them. Among the females, none of the no-service group and only 5 percent of the comparisons entered apprenticeships. An important reason for the failure of the no-service males to complete apprenticeships was their inability to cope with the academic coursework and tests required in conjunction with on-the-job training.

When we examined the kinds of jobs held by members of the study population, it was clear that the comparisons were more often in jobs requiring higher levels of skill. This was based, however, on the small percentage of male comparisons who were supervisors, journeymen, and artisans. To examine the level of job skill directly, we classified jobs according to a local modification of the Registrar General's Classification of Occupations (see Chapter 14). When we had classified each person's job history, we found that skill level was highest at age 22, so this was the age at which we examined level of job skill (Table 16.4). Among those employed at age 22, significantly more no-service males (63 percent) and females (67 percent) than comparison males (24 percent) and females (18 percent) held unskilled jobs.

Housewives. Almost equal proportions of the no-service females (40 percent) and comparison females (42 percent) were housewives. Among the no-service women, 5 percent were not employed and did not fit into the categories already described; they were not housewives and not seeking employment, but living with parents and sometimes providing some help around the house.

Take-home pay. As might be expected, take-home pay was related to level of job skill, but each level also offered a range of pay. At each level, the no-service males received significantly less take-home pay than the comparisons. Among females, the numbers at each level of skill were too small for meaningful analysis.

Subjective Measures

Reasons for leaving jobs. For every job the young people left, we asked them why they left (see Table 16.5). We also asked them which job they liked most and least, and why. Their responses clearly reflect their own evaluation of the job, not their employer's view. The reasons given fall under the general categories of the employee being fired, the job being terminated by the employer but due to no fault of the employee, or the employee having left a job of his own accord. The most frequently cited of these categories is the last.

Employee was fired. The most frequent reason the young people gave for being fired was that their behavior was unacceptable to their employer. The comparison males gave this explanation more often than the no-service male group and both female groups. When we examined the responses, we found that among comparison males, one young man gave fifteen of the twenty-two responses; among comparison females, one young woman gave three of the four responses.

Table 16.4 Level of job skill for current occupation at age 22 for no-services MR and comparisons, by gender

	Males				Females			
	No Service		Comparisons		No Service		Comparisons	
Current Occupation	*N*	(%)	*N*	(%)	*N*	(%)	*N*	(%)
Skilled employment	1	(2)	11	(33)	0		5	(45)
Semi-skilled employment	20	(36)	14	(42)	6	(33)	4	(36)
Unskilled employment	35	(63)	8	(24)	12	(67)	2	(18)
Total	56		33		18		11	
Housewife					16	(40)	8	(42)
Unemployed	4	(7)	0		4	(10)	0	
Not working, not seeking work, nor a housewife					2	(5)	0	
Overall totals	60		33		40		19	

By contrast, among the no-service young people, there was no one who gave these responses with exceptional frequency, which helps to explain the high percentages given by the comparison males. The no-service young adults, both male and female, almost exclusively reported that they were fired for being unable to cope and for lacking the skill or the physical ability to do the job. A few could give no reason why they were fired.

Jobs terminated by employer, no fault of employee. Jobs left because of termination were seasonal, being phased out, or in firms that were closing down. Among the males, job termination occurred more frequently among the no-service group than among the comparisons.

Employee left of own accord. Among no-service individuals and comparisons of both sexes, leaving of their own accord was the most frequent reason given for leaving a job. Those who offered this explanation most frequently were male comparisons (57 percent). In the different categories subsumed under "leaving of own accord," the only notable difference was among males: comparisons, more often than those in the no-service group, left in order to take other jobs or enter training programs. They usually claimed either that the pay was poor or that they disliked the job or were fed up. The no-service females left jobs because they were too physically demanding more often than the comparisons.

Table 16.5 Reasons for leaving job given by no services MR and comparisons, males and females (in percent)

	Males		Females	
Reasons for leaving jobs	No Services	Comparisons	No Services	Comparisons
Employee was fired				
Unable to cope; lacked skills, abilities, or physical requirements	4	1	6	0
Behavior unacceptable to employer	8	14	8	6
Fired, other, no reason given	2	4	1	1
Total	14	19	15	7
Job terminated by employer, but for no fault of employee	*13*	*6*	*7*	*5*
Employee left job of own accord				
Not enough pay	19	20	11	11
Disliked the physical environment at work	6	4	6	3
Job too physically demanding	2	1	6	1
Generally disliked job, fed up	13	13	12	14
Left for another job or to enter training program	6	13	3	1
Other	2	6	4	9
Total	48	57	42	39
Problems with persons in work place	8	8	10	17
Illness, accidents at and away from workplace	5	5	6	1
Pregnancy or to become a housewife	—	—	11	20
Sent to prison, other trouble with law	3	1	0	0
Other	8	4	10	11
Total number of reasons given	287	162	137	66
Number of reasons given per person	5.2	4.9	3.9	3.9

For the remaining categories, a few observations are worth noting. More than any other group, comparison females left fewer jobs because of illness or injury and more jobs because of interpersonal problems in the workplace. This finding was surprising, but when we looked into it further to see if one person was contributing unduly, such was not the case. Only males left jobs because they were sent to prison, but they do not account for all the prison sentences in the study population, only those that resulted in job loss. No-service females left fewer jobs because of pregnancy or becoming a housewife than comparison females, but this was to be expected, since fewer of them were married.

Most-liked and least-liked jobs. We examined the reasons given by the no-service group and the comparison group for liking and not liking jobs but found no differences, showing that the two groups evaluated jobs in similar ways. We will describe the results, therefore, for the no-service group only.

The reasons the study population most liked and least liked their jobs, and the frequency with which they offered a particular reason, reveals something of their job concerns (see Table 16.6). The physical conditions of the workplace were mentioned most frequently. These included negative factors such as cold, dampness, noise, smell, and

Table 16.6 Reasons given for choosing job as most or least liked by the no services MR group, by gender (in percent)

	Males		Females	
Reasons	Least liked	Most liked	Least liked	Most liked
A. Physical conditions of workplace	50	20	25	0
B. Interpersonal relations				
Workmates mentioned	0	13	9	10
Supervision mentioned	4	9	25	0
People at work (general)	0	13	0	0
Customers and clients	0	2	0	10
Total B	4	37	43	40
C. Characteristics of the job				
Interesting/boring	18	20	6	20
Variety of things to do	0	2	0	10
Autonomy given to employee	0	9	0	10
Physical demands on employee	7	4	13	0
Pay	7	2	13	10
Hours	11	4	0	5
Perks	0	2	0	5
Lack of job security	4	0	0	0
Total C	46	41	31	60
Total number	28	46	16	20

dust in the air, and positive factors such as being out in the open air, working near others so they were easy to talk to, and having comfortable working arrangements. Both sexes named unpleasant physical arrangements as reasons for liking a job least, and pleasant arrangements for liking a job most. The second most frequently given reasons were related to whether the jobs were interesting or boring. Among males, the number of positive and negative choices were balanced, but females more often referred to liking jobs because they were interesting.

The third through fifth most frequent reasons were related to interpersonal relations. Males described liking jobs most because of workmates, supervision, and people at work (in general). Females, on the other hand, offered these reasons in nearly equal numbers to describe both most-liked and least-liked jobs. Workmates and, particularly, supervision were more often mentioned as reasons for liking jobs least.

The reasons given least frequently by the study population dealt with various characteristics of the jobs themselves. Young people liked work that provided a variety of things to do as well as some personal autonomy and perks. The remaining reasons—the physical demands of the job, pay, hours, and lack of job security—are instructive in terms of employee concerns, but too infrequent to allow any reasonable conclusions about whether they deal with least- or most-liked jobs.

In the context of reasons for leaving jobs and for liking and disliking jobs, three recurrent themes appeared to be salient. The first was the physical conditions and environment of the workplace, and we examined the responses coded under these categories. For males, the conditions described most often dealt with being indoors or outdoors. Some who worked indoors felt shut in and oppressed. Others disliked inside jobs because of noise, smell, dirt, heat, cold damp, and air pollution. They wanted to get outdoors to avoid being tied down in one place. Some liked their outdoor jobs most because they were not closed in and could move about. While the majority spoke favorably of the outdoors, some also mentioned the disadvantages of being out in all kinds of weather and getting wet or cold.

A second recurrent concern dealt with supervision on the job, both negative and positive. Respondents cited too many bosses ("one person told you one thing, another told you something else"); degree of supervision ("always breathing down my neck"); whether employers showed appreciation ("they just took you for granted" or, alternatively, "it really boosts you when they say you're doing great"); and personal characteristics of the supervisor ("sarcastic," "moody," "talked religion all the time," or alternatively, "friendly," "treated workers as equals," "would lend a hand," or "would listen to you").

A third concern was the interest or boredom of the job. One of the main reasons workers left of their own accord was boredom, whereas they liked jobs with intrinsic interest.

Histories of MR Services and Jobs

Our focus thus far has been the young people with MR who received no adult services, because we wanted to consider what happened to those who disappeared from MR services after leaving school (Gruenberg 1964). To complete the picture of job histories, we will now look at the fourteen males and five females who had jobs and also received some adult MR services. We excluded an additional male and four females who had unsuccessful work trials of three months or less.

The median time the fourteen males spent out of the work force and in adult MR services was two years, and they spent more time in MR services between the ages of 16 and 18 than at other ages. Half had been in day and half in residential services. The most common career path was for them to enter the labor force after leaving school and hold a series of jobs for short periods. They then entered MR services for one to three years and subsequently reentered the labor force, with varying success, up to the age of 22. Two had a slightly different history: they remained in the work force during the years immediately after leaving school and then moved into residential services for the remaining years up to age 22.

Because time out of the work force was, by definition, greater for those who received services, we did not examine it in comparing the job histories of the males who received some services and the no-service males. On the measures of deviance based on the rates of unemployment and job turnover, the young men who received services were more deviant. With one exception, all were employed in unskilled jobs, none of which involved interpersonal relations.

The five females showed distributions similar to the males in the amount of time they spent in adult services and at what age, but there were too few of them to make any comparisons with the no-service females. In general, the young people of both genders with some time in MR services and some time in the work force experienced problems making the transition from the world of school to the world of work and needed the help of services. With two exceptions, who were male, all had left services by age 20.

Working in a Textile Mill and in Fish Processing

To better understand the daily lives of the young people in the workplace, we have selected for detailed description the two kinds of jobs in which those with mental retardation (but few comparisons) were most frequently employed: manufacturing processes at a textile mill and fish processing. "Working in the fish" was the local term for the latter and "fish houses" for the processing firms themselves, and we will use both. The descriptions of the textile and fish processing industries that follow are based on the responses given by young people during the interview, on direct observation, on talks with managers at the places of employment, and on descriptions in the official handbooks published by the city of Aberdeen.

The Textile Factory

The century-old textile manufacturing firm was located in downtown Aberdeen. At the time of the study, it produced heavy flax industrial canvas for such products as fire hoses and lorry (truck) covers. The early stages of the process produced a heavy vegetable dust, so thick that at times one end of the factory floor could not be seen from the other end. Various attempts to extract the dust with fans had been made, but these were largely unsuccessful, and it settled on the floors and machines. The processing spaces had to be kept warm and humid to maintain the flexibility of the flax, an attractive feature for workers during the winter. But the machines had a high noise level and before ear plugs were used, long-term workers suffered hearing losses.

The factory managers faced a chronic problem in obtaining unskilled workers because of the poor working conditions and gladly hired young people directly from the special school. These workers started out at age 15 or 16 as bobbin setters in the spinning room, where their task was to replace the full bobbins on the spinning racks with empty ones. Because the racks were close to the ground, being small was an advantage. The young people from the special school generally had a reputation for good attendance and punctuality, and this was attributed to parental concern and supervision. The noise level in the spinning room was lower than elsewhere in the mill, so the twelve to fourteen workers employed there could talk to one another. Bobbin setting was a repetitious job with little intrinsic interest; the only rewards were interpersonal and came from the spinners, older women who often took an interest in the young bobbin setters. The job started at very low pay, with some sort of raise every six months, but when workers reached age 18, they were eligible for a raise of 20 percent to 30 percent to meet the statutory minimum wage requirement. This was an incentive for the company to replace them with younger workers, and those that were not fired moved on to other jobs.

As young women approached the age of 18, they were tried out as machine operators in the spinning room. If they seemed promising and showed manual dexterity, they became spinners. This job consisted of watching the machines and repairing breaks in the thread. For the young men at 18, there were also various jobs available. One was barrow boy, which involved transferring parts of the manufactured product from one department to another. Another was a tenter's assistant. The tenter prepared the looms, a skilled job that required the completion of an apprenticeship; the assistant did unskilled manual jobs under the tenter's direction. There were also jobs as cleaners and laborers that involved heavy lifting and moving, such as loading the final products into trucks for transportation.

Among those from the special school, twenty-six males and nine females held at least one job at the textile factory. The majority started as bobbin setters, but others as worked as barrow boys, laborers, and cleaners. Two became tenter's assistants. Among the females one became a spinner, one collected samples for testing, and the others were cleaners.

The most common reasons workers gave for leaving the factory were the dust and dirt, but some also mentioned poor pay, being fed up doing the same job, and rows (quarrels) with gaffers (bosses). Members of the youngest cohort mentioned being laid off because machines were being changed to accommodate a move away from flax to synthetics. Most spent only short periods at the factory before leaving to try to find more attractive jobs. Only a few worked at the factory throughout the postschool period from age 15 or 16 to 22.

Fish Processing

Fish processing was carried out in a large number of local fish houses, which employed anywhere from three to over twenty people. There was considerable turnover in the unskilled jobs, especially in the smaller establishments. The young people in the study worked for ninety-seven different employers over the years from 1966 to 1977. The few larger firms occupied factories with chill rooms for freezing and packaging fish to meet the growing supermarket demand. But the small fish houses made up the majority, and these are where most of the young people in the study worked. Several of those we visited were housed under the arches that supported the railway and the two ends were enclosed by wooden partitions to keep out the elements.

The primary product in the majority of the fish houses was fish fillets, but they also processed some of the by-products into pet food. The work revolved around the filleters, a skilled job, largely learned while working in the fish houses but also taught at formal schools. Requiring somewhat less skill was skinning the fish, and this job was sometimes interchangeable with filleting. Filleting consisted of quickly but skillfully cutting the fillets to minimize loss of fish flesh. The filleters stood on wooden gratings at each side of a long table. They worked at piece-work rates, or were paid bonuses for high production, and could make a lot of money. To work efficiently, they needed a steady supply of fish prepared for filleting and a clean work space, from which the fillets, along with by-products and offal, were continuously removed.

The fish had already been gutted on the trawlers after being caught. They were packed in boxes and brought by truck to the fish house, where the fish heads were cut off and the remainder was put through a machine with small blades that removed the fins ("finning"). After finning, the fish were supplied to the filleters and skinners at their work tables, and the fillets removed and packed in various ways. Some were placed on frames, frozen, and then packed and stored in freezers. The by-products were ground up and made into pet food, which was also frozen. Sometimes by-products were sold to other specialized merchants. The final products were loaded onto trucks to be delivered to buyers. Support workers cleaned the floors and washed and sterilized the fish boxes, trays, and bowls. These were largely repetitious, unskilled jobs offering little autonomy and closely supervised. In the smaller fish houses the division of labor was less clear-cut, which gave a young person initially employed in unskilled work the opportunity to become acquainted with all phases of fish processing and a chance to learn more advanced skills.

Some of the fish houses prepared smoked fish, and this required the preparatory operations of pickling and tinting before smoking. Tasks included lighting and maintaining the fires needed for smoking, and mixing and preparing the dyes for the tinting and pickling mixtures. A few houses specialized in shellfish. Here, the equivalent of the filleter peeled the prawns or opened the shellfish. These jobs were also piecework or offered bonuses for high production. The hours of work depended on the orders in hand and the amount of fish landing at the ports. Sometimes workers had to work long hours of overtime, while at other times they had little or nothing to do.

Apart from record keeping in the fish houses, jobs did not require skills in literacy and numeracy but rather, manual dexterity and speed, and for the laboring jobs, physical strength. The young people in the study population who worked "in the fish" made numerous comments about the unfavorable aspects of the work—the cold, the dampness, working with their hands in cold water, and developing sores from the cold. In addition, certain kinds of fish produced rashes, and there were injuries from the use of knives, fish bone punctures, and being struck when stacks of fish boxes fell. Some of the jobs involved standing for long hours in one place or lifting heavy objects.

A few young people commented on things they liked about the work, which usually referred to social relationships. Some came from families who had worked in the fish for two or more generations, and some even worked in the same fish house as their relatives. The relatives were often long-time employees who knew the other older workers, which encouraged the development of a familylike relationship. Some reported that they enjoyed the conversations, the stories, the humor, and social interchange that went on around the filleting tables. The more senior workers sometimes encouraged the young people to talk about themselves and their problems, and responded with advice or help, such as lending money.

We also heard negative comments about social relationships at work. Individuals reported "wives" nagging and shouting across the tables, foul language, fighting, and a feeling that some workers were cold and inhospitable. New employees were sometimes subjected to hazing, such as a dowsing with cold water. Some had unpleasant experiences with their gaffers, or bosses, who overloaded them with work or took a dislike to them, while others reported liking their gaffers, who would lend a hand when needed and were friendly and understanding. The young people frequently moved from one fish house to another in search of steadier work, more pay, and more congenial fellow workers. The poor working conditions and low pay for unskilled people at times made it difficult for the fish houses to find help, but there was no prejudice against hiring young people from the special school.

The fish houses faced an additional difficulty in recruiting employees: stigma. The fish houses were located on the "wrong side of the tracks." Workers formed what might almost be called a subculture, many living in the same part of Aberdeen. A supervisor at one of the large fish processing plants reported that when a shopping center opened up in Aberdeen, the plant lost many women workers to the shops, even though the women took a cut in pay. He attributed this to their being attracted to jobs where they could dress well. Women fish workers would often try to hide their work clothes if they left the fish house during the lunch break. A young man in the study said he had not told his girlfriend where he worked for fear it would end their relationship. Another spoke of being ostracized on buses because he smelled of fish.

One young woman from the study explained why she took a job in the fish. When she left the special school, she wanted to work in a shop or a bakery. She applied for jobs in these places but was unsuccessful, even with the help of relatives and the youth employment service. She felt she was turned down because she had been at the special school and people thought, "You must be backward or something." Then, on her own, she got a job in the fish and told us, "It is not difficult to get into the fish if you have been to Beechwood" (the special school).

For some, having come from the special school caused problems working in the fish. A young man, in response to being asked whether anyone at work had ever teased, bullied, or made fun of him, told about working with someone he had known as a child. "He used to call me 'Beechwood' when I was a message boy in the fish, and he used to laugh at me. He told everybody and they all laughed at me. I was going to leave and the boss said not to bother." Similar teasing occurred in other jobs because he could not spell, and he would start crying. Some young people stayed in the fish because they were afraid they would not be able to find other kinds of jobs.

Summary and Conclusions

An important aspect of young adult lives is the job in which they are employed. At work, the nature of the job influences the kinds and levels of satisfaction they experience. Outside of work, the job and take-home pay influence a person's standard of living, life style, and social relationships.

In this chapter, we have focused on young people's job histories to try to determine, as Gruenberg asked, what happens to young people who were considered to have mental retardation as children but disappeared from MR services after leaving school. We considered amount of unemployment, job turnover, time out of the job market, level of job skill, take-home pay, kinds of jobs held, and some evaluation reports on how individuals felt about their jobs.

To answer the question of whether or not they are distinguishable from their peers who are not mentally retarded is more difficult. By dichotomizing the question into distinguishable or not distinguishable, reviewers have made the issue more provocative. Our findings show wide variation in job histories. The only direct way to answer the question of distinguishability would be to determine how others perceived these young people, and this we did not do. From the information we obtained, we can only make inferences based on whether there were group differences in the job histories of those who did and those who did not have MR.

Among the men, the no-service group more often held less skilled manual jobs with lower pay than the comparisons. They more often worked at laboring and cleaning jobs and less often as supervisors, salesmen, journeymen, and artisans. Fewer entered and none completed apprenticeships.

Among the women, the no-service group were out of the job market more often than the comparisons and held jobs that like the men's, required lower levels of skill, as cleaners, packers, and factory assembly line workers. They less often had jobs requiring interpersonal skills.

We also obtained some measures of how individuals rather than groups differed by using deviance measures—deviance defined as being in the lowest 10 percent of the distribution of scores of the comparisons—for unemployment, job turnover, and time out of the job market. Of the no-service men, 26 percent were deviant on one of the measures, and a further 7 percent on two or three of the measures, while the percentages for women were very similar.

Although we have described the group differences between the no-service and the comparison young adults, to provide a balance it is important to emphasize that on some measures, some of the no-service group functioned as well as many of the comparisons. Just over one third of the no-service group held semiskilled jobs, and 20 percent held jobs requiring interpersonal skills. Two thirds of the no-service group were not deviant on any of the three deviance measures. There were no differences in rates of job turnover between the no-service and the comparison groups.

We have the clear impression that the impairments of literacy, numeracy, and language that caused the no-service group to be classified as mentally retarded in childhood still remained for many of them and made them distinguishable from others.

We initially developed the category of jobs requiring interpersonal skills as a way of looking at social competence but found that they also required reading, writing, and dealing with numbers. Thus, a receptionist takes phone messages and makes appointments, a bus conductor must charge the correct fares for journeys of different lengths and make change, and a shop assistant (store clerk) has to deal with money and keep and refer to written records. The differences between the number of individuals with MR who received no services and comparisons employed in jobs requiring interpersonal skills may have been due to a lack of literacy or of competence with numbers, as well as a lack of interpersonal skills—or all three. Indeed, the results for those who received no MR services suggest that a major obstacle in applying for and holding jobs was a persistent lack of literacy and numeracy. These skills were needed, especially in the off-the-job training given during apprenticeships and in the certification process. (It was a greater problem for females than for males, because female comparisons—significantly more often than male comparisons—had jobs requiring interpersonal skills.) Lack of skills in literacy and numeracy prevented some of the no-service group from advancing to more skilled jobs. For example, many of the comparisons, as a first job, became delivery boys, working under the supervision of the van driver, a job they held only to age 18, when employers had to pay a considerably higher statutory minimum wage. Among the comparisons who started as van boys (drivers' helpers), some became van drivers because they obtained a driver's license and were able to do the paperwork and reading required for the job. Almost without exception, however, the no-service group were unable to pass the written part of the driver's test, and even if they had, would not have met the literacy requirements for a van driver. While a number of comparison women had waitress jobs, no one in the no-service group was able to function as waitress. Some worked in cafes and restaurants as dish washers and cleaners, and a few had unsuccessful trials as waitresses. They reported that they could not cope with taking orders and keeping them straight, or the interpersonal relations with customers.

A number of the young people indicated that they were only too aware of their academic shortcomings and would have liked further opportunities to learn to read, write, and use numbers. The special school for children with MR had evening classes on these subjects for former pupils, and a number of our subjects took advantage of the offerings. It is more difficult to assess the extent to which limited skill in conceptual thinking, adaptive behavior, or social competence also create obstacles for young people with MR in their job careers. Even in jobs that do not require these skills, young people reported being teased and bullied when it was found out that they were unable to read or write or had difficulty in doing so.

In addition to the no-service group who disappeared from MR services after leaving school, some young adults who spent most of their time in the job market also received some adult MR services. If these were added to the no-service group, the combined groups would do less well in their job histories than the no-services group alone.

We restricted the comparisons to those who left school without the academic qualifications needed for further education and more skilled jobs because no one with MR had those academic prerequisites. Had we included the comparisons who left school with academic qualifications, the differences between them and the no-service group would have been far greater.

As we have pointed out, one reviewer (Rosenbrock 1985) suggested that workers with MR would not mind the repetition and tedium of industrial jobs. Our results show that they disliked these jobs just as frequently as the comparisons. More generally, individuals with MR resembled comparisons in their reasons for liking or disliking jobs.

The results suggest that the no-service group, especially the men, had less control over their working lives than the comparisons. The men in the no-service group more often left a job because it was terminated by the employer, it was seasonal, or the firm went out of business; they less often left jobs of their own accord. The no-service group more often left jobs because they were unable to cope with the work and less often in order to go to another job or to get training. This suggests that the no-service group may have had more difficulty in planning for job changes, and with fewer skills to offer, may have had more difficulty in finding new jobs. Their higher rate of unemployment provides some evidence for this. Many of the no-service men were able to succeed in finding new jobs because they accepted poor working conditions and low pay.

Approximately two-thirds of the no-service group held unskilled manual jobs. These were often repetitious and of little intrinsic interest, located in unpleasant physical environments, and offered little or no autonomy or responsibility in organizing the work. Under these conditions, pleasant social relationships in the workplace were the only possible redeeming feature. A key element was the supervisor, who had the power to make working conditions pleasant or unbearable.

In the small fish processing plants, workers stood around a common work table, which encouraged social interaction. More directly, stable employees, a benevolent head of the firm, and older workers who took an interest in the young people doing the unskilled manual jobs contributed to congenial interpersonal relations and made a boring and uninteresting job agreeable.

A young man in the no-service group who worked for the city as the junior member of a team of three on a garbage truck cited this as his most liked job. The team members had a daily quota but could organize the work as they wished, which allowed them to set their own pace and arrange for times to stop for lunch or a cup of tea. The two senior members of the team treated the junior well and there was plenty of time for talk.

It is of interest that the young men in the no-service group most often mentioned interpersonal relations in connection with jobs they liked most. By contrast, the young women gave this as the reason they liked jobs most and least with almost equal frequency. This may be related to gender differences in the kinds of jobs held; 70 percent of the women worked either in division of labor jobs or as packers. Both types usually involved assembly lines (where men worked less often), which appeared to have closer and more impersonal supervision. Most of the supervisors were men, some of whom had little understanding of the needs of women, and some of the women spoke of sexual harassment.

Because interpersonal relations are so important in unskilled manual jobs, further study of how to organize work in order to encourage productivity and job satisfaction and make the workplace more congenial is essential. Our results do not directly answer the question of whether those who disappeared from MR services were distinguishable in their job histories from peers who did not have MR. It is reasonable to infer that some clearly were, and that only a minority were not distinguishable.

17

Activities outside Working Hours

One of the central concerns of the present study has been the adjustment of young adults with mild mental retardation (MR) to adult life. In this chapter we will look at how they spent their nonworking hours during evenings and weekends for the period around age 22, including the time they devoted to leisure activities and to carrying out their responsibilities and obligations (housework, child care, and overtime hours or extra jobs). Cutting across all of these activities are the various forms of social relationships so crucial to the lives of these young adults.

The chapter will focus primarily on the young adults with mild MR who were not receiving adult MR services, although we will also consider young adults with mild MR who were in day services in the community. We have excluded from our analysis those who were living in residential institutions and those with severe MR because their lives were generally circumscribed, restricted, and supervised.

To illustrate the great diversity in the study population we present several case histories. The first two reveal social isolation and the paucity of leisure activities.

Neil lived with his parents, but his father was often away for long periods because of his job. Neil spent most weekends by himself watching TV, listening to the radio, and looking at the newspaper. Because he worked an evening shift, Neil was prevented from participating in many leisure activities, so that socializing was difficult. He had joined a cycle club but lost interest after his bike was stolen. He had also tried a judo club, but his work hours complicated his attendance at classes and he withdrew after he hurt his shoulder. He was interested in electronics and tried reading an electronics magazine, but he had difficulty with big words. Neil had never had a girlfriend, and he had no close friends. Occasionally, he went alone to a hotel where there was dancing in hopes of meeting a girl, but because he was shy and could not dance, he was always unsuccessful. He described himself as "not much of a conversationalist" and said that he did not talk to anyone. If he felt his company was not needed, he disappeared. When asked what advice he would give to others about finding a girlfriend, he replied, "If you are no good at it yourself, how can you give advice?" He always seemed to get on better, he thought, when he was alone. Asked about qualities that might make him a poor husband, he replied, "By being lonely, I don't go out much, don't have many friends. Maybe I'm a bit of a bore."

Janet also lived with her parents. On weekends she slept late and spent a lot of time alone watching TV or listening to tapes and records. She like to read the newspaper to see if she knew any of the brides in the wedding announcements. She was one of seven children, and her siblings lived nearby. She saw them fairly frequently but did not feel close to any of them. Some evenings or weekends she went to her brother's house and looked after the children when he and his wife went out. She also did some sewing and sometimes played cards with one of her brothers or went into town with her mother, but she had no other interests she thought she would like to pursue. She said she did not feel close to anyone and did not want any close relationships. People found it difficult to understand her speech, and this may have complicated social interaction. She liked being alone because when she was with people she started trouble, and she was afraid she might hit them. At one time Janet had a job in fish processing, but she stopped when she was told it was bad for her health. After that, she stayed home and helped her mother with the housework.

Two other case histories indicate a more extensive set of social relationships, interests, and activities.

Stephen had been married for about a year, and his wife was pregnant with their first child. Before their marriage, they rarely went out, because they were saving money to furnish a home. He helped his wife in their flat, but she did the cooking and shopping. On Saturday mornings he worked, and in the afternoon he usually played soccer, one of his favorite activities. He had difficulty reading, but looked at the sports pages of the newspaper. At work, sports were a major topic of conversation. His other favorite activity was making models from kits and painting them. Stephen and his wife often watched TV in the evening or listened to records and tapes of popular music, which they collected. Sometimes they went out to the movies. Before his wife became pregnant, they enjoyed swimming. Stephen had an active social life. On his own he went to visit friends, and they would go for a drink at the pub. He and his wife were friendly with another couple, and the four of them often spent Friday evenings at each other's homes, and they enjoyed arguing about politics. At other times, they went for walks or to the beach. They were also very friendly with neighbors. Stephen had friends from work and other friends he had met when he was active in a boys' club. He belonged to two social clubs, one where he went after work for a drink, and the other where he and his wife went dancing. Stephen and his wife both had parents and siblings living nearby, whom they visited. Stephen said that since his marriage, he felt he had more responsibilities but that nothing else had changed.

Sheila was single and lived with her parents. She was part of a closely knit extended family and named her grandmother and an aunt as two of her three best friends. There was considerable visiting within the extended family, and Sheila talked about her cousin's engagement party, when many family members had gathered for drinks and dinner. She had many friends at work, and they went out together every week or two. They hired a minibus and went to different places for drinks and dancing. One of her friends from work was a best friend, and they visited each other's homes, or went out together every week. Sheila was close to her parents and went with them when they visited friends or for a ride in their car. She helped her mother with the housework. Recently, Sheila had been attending church and taking classes given by the minister. She enjoyed the church music. Sheila also took a course in dressmaking and enjoyed making clothes. She liked going out for walks, going to the movies with a friend, and skating. She said she had no problems with reading and read the local paper to keep up with the happenings in Aberdeen.

We obtained full information about activities and social interactions outside of working hours from 85 young adults with mild MR who were not receiving services and 88 nonretarded peers (comparisons). Data on leisure-time activities were taken from a section of the interview in which the young adults were asked to describe how they had spent the previous weekend, from five o'clock on Friday evening through Sunday evening, and how they had spent the previous weekday evening. Interviewers asked probing questions to obtain full coverage of the time periods and to clarify and expand unclear or brief responses. The young adults were also asked to describe how other weekends might have been different from the previous one, and about seasonal differences. These open-ended questions were followed by a series of directed questions covering a wide range of leisure activities.

The interview included many questions about friends and socializing in various contexts. As the interviewer asked about particular settings, such as neighborhood, workplace, and clubs, the young adults were asked whether they had friends in that setting, what they did together, and where. They were then asked whether they still saw any of the friends they had made at school and whether they could name two best friends. If they were single, they were asked whether they had a special boy or girlfriend. If they were married, they were asked a series of questions about their spouse and children, about the marital relationship, and how well the marriage was working out.

General Measures

From a content analysis of the relevant interview data we developed seventeen categories of activities:

1. Being with other people
2. Being alone
3. Visiting or being visited
4. Participating in competitive sports
5. Doing noncompetitive physical activities
6. Reading as an intrinsic interest
7. Reading to gain particular information
8. Attending classes to further education or skills
9. Attending classes related to sports or hobbies
10. Pursuing hobbies
11. Going to pubs and hotel bars

12. Going out to organized entertainment or sporting events
13. Playing games at home
14. Playing games in clubs or pubs
15. Pursuing casual, unplanned activities
16. Choosing to do activities customarily regarded as obligations or responsibilities
17. Participating in activities out of a sense of obligation rather than pleasure.

In addition, we also developed a measure of the diversity of leisure-time activities for each person by summing scores of present (1) or absent (0) on fourteen of the seventeen leisure categories (not including time spent with others, time spent alone, and time reduced by obligations and responsibilities).Watching television was universal for all young adults, whether or not they had MR, and when we analyzed the amount of time they spent watching television and the types of programs they watched, we found no clear differences, and thus did not include television viewing as a category.

To learn more about social relationships, we developed the three following measures.

People with Whom Young Adults Spent Time

The people with whom the young adults mentioned spending leisure time were grouped in two categories, family and nonfamily, and each of these categories was subdivided by age: the older generation (age 40 and older), peers (16 to 39 years of age), and children (less than 16 years old). The resulting six categories were coded 0 for no one, 1 for one person, and 2 for two or more persons.

The analyses discussed in this chapter were first reported in Richardson, Katz, and Koller (1993, 1994) and Koller, Richardson, and Katz (1988a,b). In these papers the results of statistical analyses are presented; here, the statistics will be omitted.

Friendships and Socializing with Peers

We examined both the numbers of best friends individuals named and whether single young adults had any relationships with the opposite sex. In addition, we developed a measure of the amount of time the young adult spent socializing with their peers based on their responses to the friendship questions throughout the interview (see Koller, Richardson, and Katz 1988a for details). Here, we used three categories: *frequent,* defined as socializing at least once a month with two or more peers (that is, friends who were close in age and not family members); *seldom,* defined as either socializing with two or more peers less than once a month or with only one peer no matter how frequently; and *none,* defined as total or near total absence of socializing with peers.

Marital Status

We noted current marital status and obtained a marital history for each young adult who had ever been married. Many more comparisons than young adults with MR had married by age 22. Some of the married individuals with MR were originally matched with comparisons who were still single. In order to examine differences in marital relationships, we undertook a rematching process, which resulted in forty-three matched pairs of young adults with MR and comparisons, all of whom had been married by age 22. Among these young adults, we evaluated and rated marital relationships as follows (see Koller, Richardson, and Katz 1988b for details):

1. No evidence of unusual marital problems or discord
2. Reports of past marital problems but no problems noted at the time of the interview (which included a few individuals who had remarried following divorce)
3. Some problems and discord noted but no marked strain on the marriage evident
4. Severe problems and discord noted resulting in a strained relationship
5. Currently separated or divorced

Analysis

We will compare the young adults with mild MR who were not receiving services at age 22 to nonretarded peers (comparisons) and then present results for the young adults with mild MR who were receiving day services in the community.

Activities

Among all the young adults, those with and without MR combined, watching television was universal. Among the other categories of activities, they spent the most time in casually pursued activities, being with others, being alone, and attending organized entertainment; they spent the least time reading (either category), attending classes (also either category), and playing games at home.

In order to get a sense of the extent and types of activities in which each individual engaged, we compiled a summary of which of the fourteen categories of leisure activities described earlier were present. The totals ranged from two to twelve, with a median of seven. We divided total scores into the highest and lowest 25 percent and the middle 50 percent and found no significant difference between those with MR and the comparisons in the distributions of total scores.

Responsibilities and Obligations

The amount of time taken up by responsibilities and obligations did not differ significantly among those with MR and the comparisons, either by gender or by marital status. When the two groups were combined, however, for each marital status females spent more time in activities involving responsibilities than males (see Table 17.1).

For males, marriage without children did not increase the time they spent fulfilling responsibilities and obligations, but when they became fathers there was an increase. For females, responsibilities and obligations increased at each step, from single to married without children to married with children.

Social Relationships

We examined social relationships with peers, with the opposite sex, and with family.

Relationships with Peers

On each of the three measures—number of best friends, amount of socializing with peers, and whether they had continued friendships with schoolmates to age 22—the young adults with MR, both males

Table 17.1 Percentages of "leisure" time spent in activities involving responsibilities and obligations, by gender and marital status, for young adults with mental retardation and comparisons, combined

"Leisure" time spent in responsibilities and obligations	Single		Married/no children		Married/with children	
	M	F	M	F	M	F
None	54	29	60	12	29	0
Less than half[a]	38	65	40	82	65	36
More than half but less than all[a]	8	5	0	6	6	54
All[a]	0	0	0	0	0	10
Total *N*	102	58	20	17	34	39

a. Of available "leisure" time.

and females, had fewer social interactions than their nonretarded comparisons (see Table 17.2).

Relationships with the Opposite Sex

Marital status. None of the young adults with mild MR who were in services at age 22 and none with severe MR were married. For both males and females, fewer young adults with MR were married than comparisons (see Table 17.3). Among those with MR and the comparisons, however, a larger percentage of females were married than males. The highest rates of divorce and separation were among females with MR. In terms of either the age at which they were married or the number of children they had, there was no significant difference between those with MR and the comparisons. At age 22, most of the couples had been married two to four years and most had one or two children.

The IQ's of the young people with MR who were married were significantly higher than the IQ's of those who remained single, and those of males were significantly higher than those of females. The respective mean IQ's were 71 for married males and 65 for single males, and 67 for married females and 62 for single females.

The following analyses deal with evaluations of marriages, and for

Table 17.2 Friendships and social relationships (in percentages) among young adults with mental retardation (MR) and comparisons, by gender

	Males (n = 45 each)		Females (n = 29 each)	
Relationships	MR	Comparisons	MR	Comparisons
Number of best friends				
0	16	2	28	0
1	24	18	31	17
2	60	80	41	83
Socializing with friends				
Frequent	58	84	28	83
Seldom	22	9	38	17
None	20	7	34	0
Friends from school				
Yes	33	55	23	79
No	67	45	87	21

Table 17.3 Marital status of young adults with mental retardation not in adult MR services and original matched comparisons by gender (in percent)

	Males		Females	
Marital status	MR (n = 74)	Comparisons (n = 68)	MR (n = 46)	Comparisons (n = 44)
Single	74	44	48	30
Married	22	50	39	70
Divorced or separated	4	6	13	

these we used the rematched comparisons. In addition, because the evaluations required more information, the numbers declined.

Marital relationships. The evaluations of the marital relationships showed that females with MR experienced significantly more problems, discord, separation, and divorce than their matched comparisons (see Table 17.4). A quarter of them were separated or divorced by age 22, six times the rate for the comparison females. Although males with MR also experienced more problems than their matched comparisons, the differences were not statistically significant.

Table 17.4 Evaluation of the marriages of the young adults with mental retardation (MR) and rematched comparisons by gender (in percent)

	Males (n = 19 each)		Females (n = 24 each)	
	MR	Comparisons	MR	Comparisons
No problems or discord evident	53	79	38	71
Problems in past, none now	5	5	8	13
Some problems or discord evident	26	0	21	8
Considerable problems or discord evident	0	5	8	4
Separated or divorced	16	11	25	4

Problems in the marriages. Some marital problems stemmed from the fact that one spouse had been classified as MR. Four of the females—but none of the males—related marital problems to their histories of MR. Two of these young women expressed fears that their husbands might discover that they had been to a special school, and the other two told of their feelings of anguish or shame at the way their husbands reacted to and used this information.

The comparisons as well as the young adults with MR encountered financial, employment, and sexual difficulties, but we found these problems more often among those with MR, and more or less equally by gender. The young men and women with MR, especially the males, also lived in other people's homes rather than in a place of their own somewhat more often than the comparisons. We were surprised to find that reports of husbands' "peculiar" behavior were five times more common among the females with MR than among the comparisons. This "peculiar" behavior included such things as behaving oddly with their child, making people uncomfortable by staring at them, and burning their wife's and children's clothes when angry. More than half of the young women with MR who had experienced at least some marital discord or were separated or divorced, had had premarital pregnancies, twice the rate of their comparisons. The young women with MR also reported being physically abused by their husbands seven times more often than the comparisons. Other problems showed only slight differences and had low frequencies.

Couples with mental retardation. In three of the marriages, both partners had MR. In two cases, study subjects were married to each other. In the third case, one of the female study subjects was married to a man with MR who was not in the study. The five study subjects involved were all individually rated as having at least some problems or discord in their marriages.

In the case of one of these couples, in two years of marriage, the husband had been in prison twice and had several long periods of unemployment. His wife reported that he had been warned to stop physically abusing her by the authorities. She was cooking over an open wood fire because their gas had been cut off for nonpayment. They had one child who appeared to be poorly cared for. The interviewer remarked that the wife slapped and shouted at the child frequently and unreasonably during the interview.

The problems of the second couple were largely financial, but these were overwhelming. The husband was employed irregularly and the wife found it difficult to manage on what little money they had. Their electricity had been cut off and they were behind in their rent. Their two children appeared to the interviewer to be reasonably well cared for, but the wife was described as looking ill; she was tired and listless with dark circles under her eyes. She reported that her usual routine was to go all day without food and then visit her parents' home in the evening for something to eat. The husband said he was very unhappy and wished he had not married.

The third couple had been through at least three separations in less than three years of marriage, mainly because of the husband's outbursts of violence toward his wife. She said he had "brain-storms" when he would "go mad and hit me from one side of the room to the other." She had filed for divorce but had been convinced to try to keep the marriage together for the sake of their two children. She said they didn't agree about anything, they argued frequently, and she became depressed. Her interview responses showed remarkable ambivalence : she would "recommend marriage—it's a great life" but "I'd rather be single." Describing her husband, she said, "He's moody, but otherwise, he's perfect . . . I wish I'd known that he was moody and got [violent].” She even hoped to have two more children.

None of the comparisons, as far as we could ascertain, was married to an individual with mental retardation.

Opposite-sex relationships. Of the single young adults with MR, only 18 percent of the males and 27 percent of the females had a relationship with someone of the opposite sex. This was lower than the percentages for the comparisons—61 percent for males and 60 percent for females. The difference was statistically significant for the males and nearly so for the females.

Family relationships. There were no differences between the young adults with MR and the comparisons in the number of family members they saw frequently. When we considered marital status, we found that it was the married young adults with children who spent the most time with their families.

We also examined the relative amount of time individuals spent with family and nonfamily members. The highest ratio of time spent with family to nonfamily was for those, both males and females, who were married with children. The lowest proportion of time spent with family members was for males who were single or married without children.

Young Adults with Mild MR Attending Adult MR Day Centers

Previous studies have shown that the leisure activities of individuals with mild MR in day centers tend to be solitary, passive, and family-oriented (Reiter and Levy 1980; Edgerton and Bercovici 1976). This might be expected if their placement in services was the result of their inability to function in various age-appropriate roles, including how they used their leisure time. Our results, based on a cluster analysis of activities, are somewhat at variance with these expectations. Among the young adults in day services for whom data were available—six males and sixteen females—none of the males and only 19 percent of the females appeared in the cluster indicating social isolation as evidenced by low scores on social interaction, visiting, and going to hotel bars (lounges), and high scores on spending time alone (for details, see Richardson, Katz, and Koller 1993).

We then examined to what extent the young adults attending day centers socialized with friends outside these supervised settings and outside the four recreational clubs in the city that were designed specifically for adults with MR and other disabilities. In addition, we also wanted to know which of these friends, if any, did not have MR.

Almost 90 percent of the young adults at the day centers—the proportions were similar for males and females—regularly attended at least one of the clubs for disabled adults. (It is of interest that none of the young adults with MR who were not in adult services attended any of these clubs.) Most of those who attended the day centers (70 percent) also saw their day-center friends outside of supervised settings, but only one socialized with a nonretarded friend. This was a young man with cerebral palsy and a childhood IQ of 71. For the six-week period preceding the interview, he had been going out several times a week with a young woman volunteer at one of the special clubs he attended.

In response to the questions about friends of the opposite sex, six of the sixteen females responded that they had a boyfriend. When pressed, however, four of the six indicated that the relationship was not "serious"; the boyfriend was "just a friend" and not someone they saw socially. The fifth said she was in love, but the relationship did not extend outside the day center. The sixth not only reported that she was in love but that she and her boyfriend were discussing marriage. She further reported that she and her "best friend" visited her boyfriend in his flat one evening a week. Her mother was not aware of either the boyfriend or the best friend and said she never allowed her daughter out at night. We decided that this relationship was probably a fantasy, what Turner (1983) has termed a "normalcy fabrication," but the possibility that the relationship existed, unknown to the mother, cannot be ruled out.

Among the young men, six out of eight responded that they had a girlfriend, but three indicated that they were "just friends" and that the relationships were not "serious." The other three reported being in love, but in two cases the relationship was not pursued outside the day center and the parents were unaware of it. In only one case was there a romantic relationship and parental awareness, and this was the young man who had been going out with the club volunteer. For the other two young men and one of the young women who reported being in love, the situation may have been similar to that described for former state school residents by Birenbaum and Seiffer (1976): "A fleeting smile exchanged between residents was often . . . the basis for regarding the other as a sweetheart . . . Having a boyfriend or girlfriend was regarded as a desired status, even when love went unrequited" (p. 17).

Finally, we examined whether the young people who socialized outside of supervised settings did so on their own, or whether they were dependent on their parents to make social arrangements and provide transportation. We found that all the young men and eight out of ten of the young women who socialized in unsupervised settings did so independently.

Summary and Conclusions

Between the ages of 16 and 22, it is usual for young people to reduce the amount of time they spend with their families and increase the amount of time they spend with peers. With marriage and children, the balance between family and nonfamily swings back somewhat toward family. This general process, however, was different for the young adults with MR and for the comparisons. One of the outstanding differences was the lower frequency of peer relationships among those with MR on each of the measures, which we found for both males and females.

A number of factors may account for this difference. One is a general lack of social competence among many young people with MR. But there are also other more specific problems. Verbal communication is important in peer relationships, and the young adults with MR had less verbal competence (Chapter 10). There is also considerable evidence that an individual's social relationships may be impaired as a consequence of his or her atypical appearance, and this was more often the case among those with MR (Chapter 12). An important component of peer relationships for many young people is continuity in the friendships they establish at school, and here, individuals with MR were again at a disadvantage. The regular schools in Aberdeen were scattered throughout the neighborhoods, but there was only one special school to serve the entire city, making after-school socializing difficult. Yet without some after-school socializing, friendships may not extend beyond the school years. In addition, for some of the young adults with MR, the stigma of the special school may have limited the continuation of the friendships they formed there. Finally, we know that the young adults with MR earned less money (see Chapter 16) and thus had less to spend than comparisons, which may have restricted some activities, such as going to pubs, where young people commonly interacted with one another.

Because many more of the young adults with MR than the comparisons came from unstable families (see Chapter 14), it might be expected that they would have fewer family members to spend time with or fewer that they actually wished to see. From this it would seem to follow that they would spend less time with family members than the comparisons. The results, however, showed no difference. When we explored further, we found that the young adults with MR from unstable family backgrounds did indeed spend less time with family members than those from stable backgrounds and comparisons. However, more young adults with MR came from stable than unstable backgrounds, and when these were combined, there was no significant difference between them and the comparisons on the number of family members they saw. Comparisons also spent a greater amount of time with peers, which left less time for family members, because they had become more emancipated from their families of origin than the young people with MR.

Among both groups of young adults, those who were married with children spent more time with family members. Outside of social relationships, we found no other leisure-time differences between those with MR and the comparisons in the amount of time they spent in any specific leisure activities, the number of activities they engaged in, or the amount of time they devoted to obligations and responsibilities.

18

Fitting the Pieces Together

The elements that make up an individual's life history may be thought of as pieces in a jigsaw puzzle: when all the pieces are fitted together, the relationships between and among them as well as a comprehensive picture of the whole become apparent.

In previous chapters we have described discrete pieces of the young peoples' histories and characteristics and considered how some of them fit together. We looked at particular disabilities, for example, in separate chapters and then identified larger patterns in Chapter 11. In Chapter 8 we showed that the risk of adult behavior disturbance was increased by two factors: childhood behavior disturbance and an unstable family.

In this chapter, we propose to consider the following questions in order to assemble additional pieces of the histories of the young adults in the study population:

- How many of the children defined as having mental retardation (MR) continue to function as MR when they become young adults?
- How well can we predict which individuals will later be placed in adult MR services?
- Can we predict how well children with mild MR who disappear from MR services after leaving school will function as young adults?

- Between the ages 16 and 22, what personal characteristics are related to how well an individual functions in various adult roles?

Early follow-up studies of children with mild MR focused on finding out what happened to them after they left special education or custodial institutions. When it became clear that the more dire predictions stemming from the eugenics movement were unfounded, some studies examined the extent to which adults who disappeared from MR services after leaving school were similar to or different from peers who did not have MR. In these studies, however, investigators had little of the systematic information on their subjects' childhood histories necessary in predicting later adult functioning. Their results described numerous separate pieces of adult lives but not how they fit together, with one general exception. After World War II, vocational rehabilitation agencies wanted to be able to predict which adults with MR would benefit most from their programs, and a number of psychological studies were carried out. When Cobb (1972) reviewed this research in *The Forecast of Fulfillment,* he concluded, "Throughout the literature, it is striking that the attempt to use specific measures such as IQ scores, aptitude scores or items of biographical information as independent predictors of adaptive success has yielded at best only a low order of predictive validity." "Success or failure" he pointed out, "is not simply inherent in the nature of the individual but is the result of interactions among at least three sets of variables, the properties of the person, the environmental interventions, and the societal accommodations" (p. 1). In another review, Gold (1972) in turn gave a negative evaluation of predictive studies, noting "the monumental failure we have experienced in trying to develop valid predictors."

The four follow-up studies reviewed in Chapter 3 said little about factors related to adult adjustment. Baller (1936) suggested that women who had greater success as adults had "better personal appearance and superior training in domestic responsibilities" and that the men who were more successful had "patience with very drab work surroundings" (p. 229).

In a review of the individuals in Baller's study, Charles (1966) commented: "Successful, as compared to unsuccessful, males were likely to have acquired a skill early and worked at it continuously, probably with a large paternalistic employer like a railroad, rather than trying a variety of occupations. They were likely to have stayed in one community rather than drifting about. Successful females were likely to have learned principles of good grooming and health care early, to have married well and be working steadily" (p. 43).

Edgerton (1993) studied a group of adults who had been released from a state institution for persons with MR in an attempt to predict who would improve, who would remain stable, and who would experience a decline in the quality of their lives. His population was different and older than that in our follow-up study, and his methods were also very different. Nevertheless, Edgerton concluded, "for the most part, my predictions were worthless" (p. 197).

We have described most of the variables dealing with the childhood histories in previous chapters—family pedigree and brain dysfunction in Chapter 6, IQ in Chapter 7, behavior disturbance in Chapter 8, social class and family stability in Chapter 14, and school placement history in Chapter 15. Another childhood variable we have not yet considered is the age at which the child entered MR services.

The variables dealing with postschool histories were of two kinds. The first we called "outcomes" because they dealt with the young adult's adjustment or functioning. The outcomes were

1. *Job histories:* rate of time employed in and time out of the labor force (see Chapter 16).
2. *Diversity of leisure activities:* a summation of the different types of activities in which individuals engaged (see Chapter 17).
3. *Peer relationships:* Ratings, based on the questions about friendships in the interviews, were "frequent" (defined as socializing during leisure time at least once a month with two or more peers); "seldom" (defined as either socializing with two or more peers less than once a month or with only one peer no matter how frequently); and "none" (defined as total, or near total, absence of socializing with peers) (Koller, Richardson, and Katz 1988a).
4. *Social interaction:* This measure was a factor score comprising time spent with other people and time spent visiting inversely related to time spent alone. It is more general than peer relationships because it includes the older as well as the peer generation, and family relationships.

The second set of variables described the characteristics of the young adults: behavior (Chapter 8), speech usage (Chapter 10), appearance (Chapter 12), and self-esteem (Chapter 13).

Mental Retardation into Adulthood

We examined the administrative classification of the children in the study as mentally retarded in Chapter 4 and have some confidence that at the time these children indeed had MR. A separate evaluation of the same children by an independent team of American psychologists concluded that the administrative classification was correct. An important issue in assembling the various pieces of the study was whether all the children should be considered as having MR in the postschool period up to age 22 or whether some should no longer be thus considered.

To define mental retardation after school-leaving age, we used the World Health Organization (WHO) definition: "marked impairment in the ability of the individual to adapt to the daily demands of the social environment" (1985, p. 8). To examine an individual's ability to meet these demands, we selected four aspects of daily living: (1) social interactions, (2) peer friendships, (3) behavior disturbance, and (4) job histories.[1] To make the distinction between adequate and inadequate functioning for social interaction and job histories, we used the 90th percentile of the range of scores for the nonretarded comparisons, on the assumption that the poorest 10 percent of the nonretarded comparisons would represent inadequate functioning. For peer relations, those who had no peer relations were defined as inadequate, and for behavior disturbance, moderate to severe was defined as inadequate. (See Richardson et al. 1992 for details of the measures). For each young adult we then determined on how many of the four measures they functioned adequately.

Functioning as MR in young adulthood. We assumed that the young adults still receiving services for all, or almost all the time between

1. See Richardson and Koller (1992) for definitions of these four aspects of functioning and what was considered adequate in each; the numbers used in the chapter are extrapolated from the results reported there. *Social interaction* and *peer relations* are defined earlier in the chapter. *Adequate behavior* was defined as mild behavior disturbance or none, and the *job history* measure was made up of the percentage of time out of the labor force, and unemployed and seeking employment, and the amount of job turnover.

the ages of 16 and 22 met the WHO definition of MR. We also included those who were unable to function adequately on any of the four measures.

Functioning as MR in young adulthood uncertain. For those who were able to function adequately on one, two, or three of the four measures, the evidence seems inadequate to make any judgment on the issue.

Not functioning as MR in young adulthood. Young adults who performed adequately in all four areas may reasonably be considered to be no longer functioning as MR.

Table 18.1 shows the results of these analyses for all the young people who survived until age 22 ($n = 215$): 37 percent continued to be mentally retarded according to the WHO definition. They consist of those who were in long-term adult MR services and those receiving no, or short-term, services who were unable to function adequately on all four measures; 18 percent functioned adequately on all four measures and may reasonably be considered as no longer mentally retarded. For the remaining 45 percent who scored adequately on one to three of the functional measures, we feel the evidence is equivocal as to whether or not they are still MR as young adults.

The percentages we have given for those who are and are not mentally retarded as young adults are probably conservative estimates, because some whose measures were equivocal may belong to the two groups for whom evidence of whether or not they were MR appears

Table 18.1 Level of functioning in the post-school period, ages 16–22

Level of functioning	*N*	Percentage
Functioning at an MR level as a young adult		
a. In long term adult services	73	34
b. In short term, or no adult services, but functioning inadequately on 4 measures	7	3
Total	80	37
Evidence equivocal, functioning adequately on 1–3 measures	97	45
Evidence that young adult is no longer MR (functioning adequately on 4/4 measures)	38	18
Totals	215	100

adequate. In terms of prevalence, we can estimate that 5.6 per 1000 (80/13,842) were still functioning as MR as young adults. Clearly, it is difficult to reduce the complexity and heterogeneity of the lives of many of the young people with mild MR to the simple dichotomy of MR present or MR absent.

Predicting Use of Adult MR Services

Existing knowledge about mental retardation would lead us to anticipate that most children with severe MR (IQ <50) will require lifelong care and supervision. In the follow-up study—with one exception, a young man with Down syndrome who lived with his parents and helped in the shop—all children with IQ's below 50 went into adult MR services.

For children with mild MR, however, who will go to adult MR services and who will not is much less clear. Using simple correlations, we ascertained which elements in childhood were related to receiving adult MR services and then combined these elements into a predictive model using discriminant analysis. We employed separate predictive models for males and for females because of the many gender differences in their histories. For males, childhood IQ, behavior disturbance, brain dysfunction, and school placement correctly predicted the use of adult services for 79 percent and the nonuse of services for 87 percent. When we combined those who were and those who were not in adult services, 85 percent of the predictions were correct (see Table 18.2).

For females, the childhood variables that anticipated the use of MR services in adulthood were somewhat different and included IQ, brain dysfunction, school placement, and age at entering MR services. These correctly predicted receipt of adult services for 76.5 percent and no services for 74 percent. When we combined those who were and those who were not in adult MR services, 75 percent of the predictions were correct (Table 18.2).

When we examined the contribution of each of the different childhood variables to the predictions, the largest contributor for males was school placement history followed closely by brain dysfunction and childhood behavior disturbance; the smallest contributor was IQ. By contrast, for females, lower IQ was the major contributor, followed by school placement history; the remaining variables made only small

Table 18.2 Results of discriminant analysis to predict whether children with mild mental retardation (IQ 50+) did or did not receive adult MR services

Actual adult placement	Predicted placement		
	No adult MR service	Placed in adult MR service	*N*
Males			
Not in adult MR services	87%	13%	61
Placed in adult MR services	21%	79%	19
Females			
Not in adult MR services	74%	26%	35
Placed in adult MR services	23.5%	76.5%	17

contributions. Because IQ predicted differently for each sex, we examined the IQ distributions for males who did and did not receive services separately from those of females who did and did not receive services. For those with IQ's of 50 to 59 (the lowest among those with mild MR), more males (44 percent) than females (35 percent) disappeared from services after leaving school. Two possible explanations appear to account for this difference. First, we know from the parent interviews that some parents felt more secure about having their daughters under supervision in adult day centers than working in environments where they might be taken advantage of. Parents of sons less often voiced these concerns. Second, because males were traditionally regarded as the primary breadwinners in the family, more pressure may have been placed on them to do without adult MR services.

Predicting the Adult Functioning of Those Who Disappear from MR Services

We needed to find out whether it would be more productive to use childhood variables to try to predict a single overall measure of adult functioning or separate specific measures. To do this, we first examined whether young adults who functioned well in one aspect of their daily lives would also function well in others; that is, whether those who had more effective job careers were also more active socially and pursued a greater variety of leisure-time interests. If so, an overall measure of adult functioning would be meaningful. On the other hand, if functioning in one role was unrelated to functioning in others, then to be of any use predictive analysis should be concerned with specific aspects of adult functioning.

In this analysis we used five of the outcome measures already described: rate of time employed, rate of time out of the labor force, diversity of leisure activities, socializing with peers, and the social interaction score. Since the rate of time out of the labor force was highly correlated with rate of time employed, we used only the rate of time employed. Among the six remaining possible relationships, only time employed and social interaction were related: the more time employed, the greater the social interaction. This correlation was significant for males ($r = .32$, $p = .03$) and nearly significant for females ($r = .29$, $p = .09$). Apart from this, the separate roles in young adulthood were not related.

As we saw in Chapter 17, the daily lives of married females were greatly constricted by the responsibilities and obligations of being a housewife and mother, whereas being a husband placed few restrictions on male social and leisure activities. This difference may account for the smaller correlations for females among any of the four measures.

To explore the childhood antecedents of adult adjustment, clearly it was more reasonable to try to predict specific aspects of adult adjustment than to use a composite measure. In an earlier analysis, we attempted to predict a composite measure and obtained only a weak predictive model (Richardson and Koller 1992).

When we examined the simple correlations between childhood and adult variables, the only significant relationships were obtained with the adult measure of time out of the labor force, and this only for males. To predict time out of the labor force for males, we used the childhood variables shown to have some relationship—behavior, IQ, school career, and family stability—in a multiple regression analysis. A significant model was obtained ($p = .000$) that accounted for a variance of 43 percent. The variance describes the contribution of the antecedent measures to the outcome—that is, the amount of time out of the labor force—and this was a reasonably good prediction. The childhood measures contributing significantly to the variance were school career ($\beta = .46$), behavior ($\beta = .28$), and IQ ($\beta = .26$).

Family stability did not make a significant contribution in the context of the other measures.

We examined why males spent time out of the labor force. A few had been in prison, and some had been out because they were sick or were injured in accidents. (Because this analysis was restricted to those who disappeared from services, time out receiving services was not a factor.)

Personal Characteristics and Adjustment in Adulthood

Having put some pieces of the childhood histories together with later adult histories, we will continue to focus on those with mild MR who disappeared from services. The adult characteristics we selected were behavior disturbance, atypical appearance, speech usage, and self-esteem, expecting that these would be related to the study population's level of functioning in various aspects of their adult lives. As before, we found more significant relationships for males than for females. For males, the following relationships were significant, or nearly so: low self-esteem ($r = .35$, $p = .02$), atypical appearance ($r = .28$, $p = .06$), and poor speech usage ($r = .40$, $p = .001$), all of which were related to low scores on social interaction. Poor self-esteem was also related to low scores on peer relations ($r = .36$, $p = .01$), and behavior disturbance was related to less time employed ($r = .29$, $p = .024$).

For females, the only association was between atypical appearance and time out of the labor force ($r = .51$, $p = .002$), but it was stronger than any of the associations found for the males.

Summary and Conclusions

A major omission in the previous follow-up studies of children with mental retardation (Chapter 3) was their general failure to put numerous discrete findings together to achieve either a more comprehensive cross-sectional or a longitudinal picture. The few studies that had made some attempt were unsuccessful. Given this background, we had low expectations of how well we could predict level of adult functioning from childhood variables. Yet we did have some success. We predicted correctly, for a large majority of the children with mild MR, who would and who would not receive adult MR services. We could have anticipated all the childhood predictors—IQ, brain dysfunction, history of childhood MR services, age at entering MR services, and behavior disturbance—although these variables had different weight for males and females (for females, IQ was more important). These variables, however, have not previously been used for predictive purposes.

Because so little is known about the lives of young people who disappear from MR services after they leave school, we were particularly interested in whether we could predict how they functioned as young adults using measures of their childhood histories. We were generally unsuccessful except in predicting how much time the young men spent out of the job market between the ages of 16 and 22, which we were able to do even though time out of the job market did not include being in adult MR services. It is of interest that the measure of family stability in childhood, although powerfully associated with adult behavior disturbance, was not a predictor of functioning in the various adult roles. In addition, throughout the analyses, relationships between pieces of the histories were stronger for males than for females.

Conclusion: Relevance of Research Findings for Today

Do the results of our longitudinal research apply only to the particular study, or do they have more general application and remain relevant today? In this chapter we address this question and summarize those findings that still apply today, those where conditions have changed, and those that are unique to our study and about which we have no basis for comparison.

There are two ways in which we may consider whether the results we obtained still apply. One is to compare our findings with those of other researchers. The other is to identify societal expectations for young people which are based on long-term customs and beliefs and have remained unchanged since the time of our study. These are described in Chapter 2 and may be broadly summarized as follows. First, children's primary involvement is with their families. In the transition to adulthood it is expected that these attachments will shift to people outside the family, especially to peers and opposite sex relationships. Second, as children grow up they are expected to assume responsibilities for managing their own affairs and become economically independent; this coincides with the change in role from student to employee. We examined the extent to which the young people with mental retardation (MR) in our study met these expectations, and it is reasonable to expect that young people with MR now will be similar in the way in which they meet the same challenges.

Findings That Still Apply

Severe Mental Retardation

Prevalence. To plan services for children and adults with MR requires information about the frequency of MR in the general population, the frequency and severity of other disabilities they may have, and the number of individuals to be served at different ages. Previous research has shown that the prevalence of severe MR has fluctuated around 4 per 1000 in childhood for at least the last fifty years, with no indication of a long-term upward or downward trend (see Chapter 5). The most recent published study of prevalence was carried out in Atlanta, Georgia (Murphy et al. 1995). In that study, the administrative prevalence rate for severe MR was 3.6 per 1000 for 10-year-old children in the period 1985–1987. This is very close to our rate of 3.3 per 1000 at the same age but obtained at a different time and in a very different community. In our study, the age-specific prevalence was relatively stable from 5 to 22 years, declining slightly as a result of mortality (Chapter 5). We also found that 30 percent had moderate to severe behavior disturbance, 22 percent had epilepsy, all had moderate to severe verbal communication disabilities, and 23 percent had cerebral palsy. These results, too, came within the range of results of other studies (see Chapter 11).

Factors causing increases and decreases in prevalence appear to balance out over time. Advances in neonatology, for example, have resulted in the increased survival of very low birthweight babies, who are at high risk of brain dysfunction. Offsetting this are advances in the care of newborns and the use of amniocentesis followed by termination of pregnancies, which have reduced the numbers of children surviving with brain dysfunction.

Social class. Social class provides some indication of the lifestyle of a family and is based on a classification of the parents' occupation, which is related to parental education and income. It is used to see how a disorder is distributed in a population. One of the most replicated results in the epidemiology of MR is that severe MR is randomly distributed across social classes, with some studies finding a slight increase at the lower end of the distribution. Our results were in accord with the general finding (see Chapter 14).

MR services and parents' burden of care. It is understood that adults with severe MR are unable to meet societal expectations for the transition from childhood to adulthood, and they usually need lifelong care and services. With one exception, all the adults with severe MR in our study received services, and their paths varied (see Chapter 15), providing useful indications of the diversity of services needed. The need for residential services is related to the stability of the families and the degree of behavior disturbance among the young people. We found that the parents' burden of caring for children with severe MR varied widely. For some of the young adults whose only additional disability was in verbal communication, the parental burden of care was relatively light. Some young people provided companionship for their parents, helped with housework, and were included in many of their parents' social activities. Some of these parents spoke of the rewards as well as the problems they had experienced with their child. (See, for example, the case study of Kathleen in McLaren 1988.) For other children with severe MR, more serious disabilities—especially severe epilepsy and behavior disturbance—made the burden of care so heavy that their parents were unable to have any recreation or social life; they had little time for each other or for other children, they suffered from chronic loss of sleep, and when they were finally no longer able to cope, they placed their child in residential care. It is reasonable that the diversity in the histories of individuals with severe MR found in our study will still be found today.

Mild Mental Retardation

Prevalence. We obtained a cumulative prevalence rate for mild MR of 12.7 per 1000 using an administrative definition and 9.4 per 1000 when only children with IQ's of 50 to 69 were included. Our cumulative prevalence is the number of children who were classified as MR at any time up to age 15. The age-specific prevalence of mild MR varied widely, increasing sharply between ages 5 and 9, changing little from 10 to 14, dropping by over a half around school-leaving age, and then remaining relatively stable between ages 15 to 22 (Chapter 5). The same pattern of age-specific prevalence was found by Gruenberg in a review in 1964. Because of these changes with age, it is important to take age into account when comparing studies. We made an age-specific comparison with the Atlanta study, where an administrative definition was also used (Murphy et al. 1995). Its prevalence rate of 8.7 per 1000 for 10-year-old children was almost identical with ours at that age. Many factors make it difficult, however, to compare prevalence rates of mild MR from different studies. In communities with very low prevalence rates for MR we would expect the drop at around school-leaving age to be less than in other studies, owing to their exclusion of many higher-functioning children at the upper end of the range of mild MR in their prevalence rate. In Chapter 5 we discussed what may have accounted for the much lower prevalence rates found for children with mild MR in Sweden. Factors affecting their results included an upward drift in IQ's, a definition of mild MR based only on IQ (with an upper limit of 70), and the difficulties researchers had in being able to identify all children whose IQ's were between 50 and 69. An upward drift increases IQ's and reduces the number of children with IQ's between 50 and 69 compared with the number that would have been obtained using an IQ test standardized with a mean of 100. These difficulties stemmed from restrictions on using IQ tests and the reluctance of educational authorities to classify children as mentally retarded. The history of how mild MR has been defined reveals a continuing difficulty in establishing the upper end of the IQ range for MR. At different times it has been placed at 70, 75, and 80, and this creates a troublesome borderline area. The present upper cutoff point is an IQ of 70, but some children with higher IQ's may reasonably be considered to have MR. Because of this uncertainty, wherever possible we compared the histories and characteristics of young people with IQ's of 60 to 69 and 70 to 79 in our study. In general, the similarities far outweighed the differences. It should be noted, however, that when we examined the proportion of all children in the city in the same birth cohorts with IQ's of 60 to 69 and 70 to 79 we found, as might be expected, that far fewer children from the total population with IQ's of 70–79 had been classified as MR than children in the 60–69 range. These findings suggest that there are children who may need special attention and help in school but who are now overlooked because they are not included in current definitions of MR.

Social class. Our study and many others before and since have found that mild MR is heavily overrepresented at the lower end of the social scale (see Chapter 6). It is reasonable that this social class distribution will continue to be found.

Societal expectations. There was wide variability in the extent to which young adults with mild MR were able to conform with societal expectations. Approximately a quarter received adult MR services, and we considered this clear evidence of their being unable to meet the general expectations of society. For the remaining young adults who received no services, an important issue we examined was how well they were able to carry out adult roles. To varying degrees we found that they had functional limitations that made it difficult for most of them to conform (Chapter 18).

Our finding that young people with mild MR in our study more often had unskilled jobs than the nonretarded has been noted in previous studies (see Chapter 3).

Our findings agreed with those of Koegel and Edgerton (1984) that the limitations in reading, writing, and numerical calculation that trouble individuals with MR at school continued to be problems for them as young adults. We found, more specifically, that these problems proved a major obstacle to better jobs. Because the young adults in our study could not pass the written test for a driver's license, they were unqualified for driving jobs; they were unable to obtain jobs requiring completion of apprenticeships because success required passing written examinations. The young women with mild MR in our study generally preferred working in an office, as a shop assistant, or as a waitress to most industrial jobs, but they were unable to cope with these preferred jobs because of poor literacy and numeracy.

These limitations helped keep two-thirds of the young adults with mild MR at the lowest level of unskilled employment, in contrast with more than three-quarters of the comparisons who held semiskilled and skilled jobs. Even at the same general level of skill, those with MR received less take-home pay (see Chapter 16). This difference in level of job skill has also been noted in previous studies. Because they had less money than their nonretarded peers, they were also less able to afford to go to pubs, hotel lounges, and similar places where young people congregated for social purposes.

Because employment was such an important part of the lives of these young adults, we asked them why they left a particular job and what kinds of work they liked and disliked. The reasons they gave suggest that individuals with mild MR have less control over their working lives than those who do not have MR. They tended to hold less secure marginal jobs and more often felt unable to cope with the work. They also left employment of their own accord less often than did the comparisons (see Chapter 17).

Their reasons for liking and disliking jobs were similar to those of the nonretarded comparisons. They *did* mind tedious, repetitive work but often could find no alternatives. Many of the jobs they held were repetitious, had little intrinsic interest, offered little or no autonomy or responsibility in organizing tasks, and were often located in an unpleasant physical environment. At the same time, supervisors had the power to make the daily lives of these workers anything from pleasant to unbearable. An important factor was the extent to which the physical location of other workers encouraged social interaction; opportunities to form congenial social relationships with workmates could make a job more attractive. It is reasonable to expect that these findings have relevance for young people today who have mild MR, who are not receiving services and are attempting to conform with societal expectations.

Other functional limitations occurred more frequently among young adults with mild MR than among nonretarded peers. These included limitations in verbal communication and social skills, which resulted in fewer nonfamily relationships and friendships with peers and thus more social isolation. In addition, fewer of those with MR were married, and those who were, especially the females, experienced more marital problems than the comparisons.

Reasons for residential placement. We found two major reasons why young people with all levels of severity of MR were placed in residential facilities. One was behavior disturbance that caused severe management problems for parents. The other was the breakdown in the family structure through parental death, separation, divorce, imprisonment, or mental illness. Neither of these reasons is specific to the time and place of our study.

Findings Where Conditions Have Changed

Changes have been taking place in the way people with MR and their place in society are viewed. Some of these changes were occurring during the time period of our study and have continued since then.

Education

An important change has been the recognition that classifying children as MR and establishing segregated services for them may have stigmatizing consequences and actually restrict their opportunities to gain the experience they need to function effectively as adults. As a result, not only have MR services become less segregated, but changes have also been put in place to try and make the lives of those with MR as normal as possible within their communities. It is perhaps natural that when changes are made in services, the more favorable aspects of the new services are emphasized, while the more negative aspects of the old forms of services receive attention. Because we examined segregated special education for children, we were able to assess some of the benefits and disadvantages it provided and gain a perspective to assess some of the consequences of the changes in the educational systems that have occurred.

In segregated special education, being with other children who had also experienced failure and stigma in regular classes and having the benefit of small classes and specially trained teachers reduced stress. At the same time, as we have suggested, students paid a price for having been segregated in a special school and needed additional help in developing skills in interpersonal relationships. They might also have benefited from more social interactions with nonretarded children, which would have been possible if they had attended a special class within a regular school. Their special placement marked them, and in later years some were stigmatized by employers, peers, and spouses to the point that they tried to conceal their special placement history. Outside of school, they were often socially isolated during childhood, an experience intensified for those from unstable families.

With the advent of normalization and mainstreaming, and the growing awareness that an MR classification can have stigmatizing consequences, there has been a move away from segregated education. It has been less well recognized that mainstreamed children are often socially isolated by schoolmates and sometimes their special educational needs left unmet because of overburdened teachers who are unfamiliar with the special needs of those with intellectual impairments. Mainstreaming can, in some ways, be as stigmatizing for a child as segregation in a special school and potentially more stressful. So far there have been no studies that have followed mainstreamed children with mild MR to see how well they fare as adults. The best educational arrangements for children may be somewhere between the alternatives of segregation and mainstreaming, but this is an issue that remains unresolved.

Adult Day Services

In Aberdeen there was originally only a single program of day services. It eventually became clear that a single program could not adequately serve adults with profound MR and multiple disabilities as well as those with mild MR who could benefit from vocational training. In time, several programs designed to accommodate the needs of a variety of adults with mild and severe MR were initiated. From the young adults in our study we learned that MR service providers also need to be sensitive to gender differences in terms of both the kinds of programs they offer and the preferences of those they serve and their families.

Residential Services

At the time of the study, adult residential care had begun to move away from the single traditional institution serving a wide geographic area and toward smaller community-based residences tailored to meet a variety of needs. As this trend has continued, increasing attention is being paid to encouraging resident participation in activities previously available to and used only by nonretarded persons, to involving residents in decision making about housing and community programs, and to encouraging residents to manage their own affairs to whatever extent they are able.

Funding Priorities

In Aberdeen, at the time of our study, a high priority was placed on human services to meet the needs of children and adults. As a consequence, these services were well funded and the standards of services were high. With few exceptions, the services that children and adults with MR needed were widely available and paid for from government revenues. In the transition from children's to adult services there were few who experienced gaps in their service needs.

In many places today this situation has changed, and lack of funds and unwillingness to increase taxes are resulting in budget cuts. Human services in general and education in particular are being given a lower priority, and this is taking a toll on children with special needs. Because of the conditions prevailing at the time of our study, the services available to our study population provides some indication of the needs of those with MR and their families. The absence of supportive services for parents whose children need extensive care will, in some cases, create an intolerable burden, leading to an inability to cope with the family situation and an emergency need to find other forms of care for the child.

Technology

New technology since the study has led to changes in the workplace. There appears to be a reduction in the number of jobs requiring unskilled manual labor. At the same time, however, technology has led to the simplification of some tasks. It is unclear how these shifts will increase or decrease the kinds of jobs that adults with mild MR will be able to perform and whether the job conditions will become more or less congenial for them.

Transportation

In Aberdeen, none of the young adults with MR was able to pass a driving test, and this precluded their personal use of cars for transportation. Because a good public transportation system existed, the absence of a car was not a serious obstacle to getting about. In communities where the quality of public transportation is poor, young adults with mild MR who are not placed in adult MR services will be at a serious disadvantage in securing a job that requires them to travel to and from work. It will also make shopping and any kind of social life with peers more difficult. There is some social status in owning a car, which they also miss.

Findings Unique to Our Study

We carried out several analyses that are unique to our research. This precludes comparison of the results with other studies, so we have no basis for determining the relevance of these issues today. We hope that future studies will address these questions.

Etiology

In Chapter 6 we examined clues to the etiology of MR using categories that have been used by others: biomedical factors, including genetic disorders, and psychosocial adversity. We added a third category, separated from genetic disorders, of intergenerational genetic disorders, the best known of which is the fragile-X syndrome; we called these disorders "family pedigree" (see Chapter 6). We determined the frequency of each of these three factors as they occurred singly and in combination among individuals with severe and mild MR. For severe MR, our results agreed with other studies that biomedical factors played a predominant causal role. For mild MR, biomedical factors were found in one-third of the children, and several recent studies have had similar findings. Family histories indicating psychosocial adversity were present for 45 percent of the children, but these occurred in combination with family pedigree or biomedical factors, or both, more than half of the time. Only 22 percent of the children with mild MR experienced psychosocial adversity alone. Because not all children who experience psychosocial adversity have MR, we may speculate that when psychosocial adversity occurs together with genetic predisposition to be at the low end of the range of intelligence, mild MR can result, and that this combination existed among those children for whom psychosocial adversity was the only factor present. To the extent that this is true, programs aimed at reducing children's experience of psychosocial adversity "may eliminate some cases of mild mental retardation, [but] the phenomenon will never be eradicated if it is part of the normal expression of the population gene pool" (Zigler 1995).

Stability and Change

For three variables—IQ, behavior disturbance, and epilepsy—we examined the degree of stability and change within the age span of our study for each individual. We also examined the continuation of MR into adulthood.

The IQ of each child showed little stability during the earlier school years, the time when most children with mild MR were classified, and the changes were more often decreases than increases in scores. It was not until the later school years that stability in IQ's became the rule, rather than the exception (Chapter 7).

Behavior disturbance was examined for stability and change between childhood and young adulthood. Half the young people had no behavior disturbance in either age period, and a quarter had behavior disturbance in both periods. The remainder had behavior disturbance in one or the other of the two age periods. A child with behavior disturbance was at greater risk of adult behavior disturbance than was a child without behavior disturbance, and the risk of continued disturbance was greatest for children with conduct disorders (Chapter 8).

Most epilepsy developed during the first two to three years of life, but new cases continued to occur up to age 20. We examined rates of remission, defined as being seizure-free for five years with or without medication. By age 22, 39 percent had attained remission. The duration of epilepsy was related to the severity of disability due to epilepsy (Chapter 9).

An important question raised by Gruenberg in 1964 and not answered since that time is whether children with MR who do not receive adult MR services continue to function as mentally retarded in adulthood or if they become indistinguishable from peers who do not have MR. The American Association on Mental Retardation (1992) emphasized that the designation of MR applies only at the time of diagnosis and should not be presumed to be a lifetime state. This caution applies essentially to mild MR. Using measures of functioning among the nonretarded comparisons, we determined adequacy in four aspects of adult life, defined as a level of functioning reached by 90 percent of the comparisons. Adults with MR who did not receive MR services and were found adequate on all four measures were no longer considered to be functioning as mentally retarded; 18 percent met these conditions. Those who were inadequate on all four adult aspects of functioning were considered to still have MR; over one-third met this criterion. For the remaining half of the young adults who were adequate on only some of the measures, it was equivocal whether they should still be considered to have MR (Chapter 18).

Family Stability

We found that 9 percent of the children with MR could not be assigned a social class. Some came from broken homes and had been brought up by several different caretakers, in foster homes, and other forms of care. Others had remained with parents who were chronically unemployed, disabled, or disordered and had no job histories. None of the nonretarded comparisons came from families for whom social class could not be assigned. The measure we developed of family stability provided more information about families than social class and was useful as an indicator of the degree of psychosocial adversity experienced during childhood. Using the scale of family stability we found that 45 percent of the children with MR and 5 percent of the nonretarded comparisons came from unstable families (Chapter 14).

Appearance

There is strong evidence from previous research that atypical physical appearance places a child or adult at a disadvantage in social intercourse. There have been no studies that examine different kinds of atypicalities. In Chapter 12 we examined various aspects of atypical appearance, including atypicalities of facial characteristics, body proportion, movement, expression, and manner. In general, we found that atypical appearance increased as IQ decreased. We examined whether those least likely to appear atypical, the young adults with mild MR who had disappeared from MR services, were more atypical in appearance than nonretarded peers. As a group they were, although almost 60 percent were either not at all atypical or they had only one minor atypicality.

Prediction

We investigated how well measures derived from childhood histories and personal characteristics would predict later adult functioning. As a first step, we attempted to predict which children with mild MR did and did not receive adult MR services. (All children with severe MR were placed in adult services.) We predicted correctly for about three-quarters of both males and females. School placement histories predicted for both. For males, however, evidence of brain dysfunction and behavior disturbance were also significant predictors, whereas, for females, IQ was the only other predictor. For the children who were not later placed in adult services, we examined what factors predicted why some functioned better than others as young adults. Because we found that adults who performed adequately in one adult role did not necessarily do well in others, we tried to predict how well they functioned in specific aspects of adult life. Our only success was in predicting the amount of time males spent out of the labor force. The childhood variables of school placement history, behavior disturbance, and IQ were significant contributors to and accounted for 43 percent of the variance (Chapter 18). Identifying characteristics of children with mild MR that predicted receipt of adult services is the only important contribution we have made to help answer parents' questions about what will happen to their children when they grow up.

Looking Back and Looking Forward

We were fortunate to have found an auspicious set circumstances in Aberdeen, Scotland, for the study of children with MR and their follow-up to age 22. These circumstances enabled us to base the study on a total representative population of children with all degrees of severity of MR. This was the first study of its kind, one that provided us with an opportunity to be comprehensive in scope. Our previous study publications dealt with particular subjects, often unrelated to one another, and this book ties them together. It may no longer be possible to carry out this kind of study because of the many changes in values related to MR and the resulting changes in the organization of services.

The term *mental retardation* and the alternative terms used may imply to some people a single disorder or condition and can encourage the stereotypical conception that MR is always associated with severe intellectual impairment, often accompanied by other disabilities. This view is partially due to the frequent atypical appearance of children and adults with severe MR in institutional settings and more recently of adults in day-care programs. One of the central points we have tried to emphasize in reporting this research has been the enormous diversity in the personal characteristics and histories into adulthood of the children who met the definition of mental retardation. We have tried to convey this diversity in both the quantitative analysis and the illustrative descriptions. We have devoted considerable attention to those about whom least is known: the approximately one-half of all the children classified as mentally retarded who after leaving the special school managed to live without receiving any adult MR services.

This study has provided us with an opportunity to investigate a series of topics that are only possible to pursue in longitudinal research. We hope that our efforts will encourage investigators and the funding sources on which they depend to carry out further studies along some of the paths we have followed.

References

Abbeduto, L. 1991. Development of verbal communication in persons with moderate to mild mental metardation. *International Review of Research in Mental Retardation,* vol. 17. New York and London: Academic Press.

Abramowicz, H. K., and S. A. Richardson. 1975. Epidemiology of severe mental retardation in children: Community studies. *American Journal of Mental Deficiency* 80, 18–39.

Adams, G. R. 1977. Physical attractiveness research. *Human Development* 20, 217–239.

Ad Hoc Consultants on Mental Retardation. 1977. *Report to the Directors of NICHD, NIH and the NIMH of the Dept. of Health, Education and Welfare.* Federal Research Activity in Mental Retardation: A Review with Recommendations for the Future.

Akesson, H. O. 1986. The biological origin of mild mental retardation: A critical review. *Acta Psychiatrica Scandinavica* 74, 3–7.

American Association on Mental Retardation. 1992. *Mental Retardation Definition, Classification, and Systems of Supports.* 9th ed. American Association on Mental Retardation, Washington, D.C.

American Psychiatric Association. 1987. *Diagnostic and Statistical Manual of Mental Disorders,* 3rd ed., rev. Washington, D.C.

Anastasi, A. 1968. Psychological Testing. 3rd ed. Ontario, Canada: Macmillan/Collier-Macmillan.

Annegers, J. F., J. D. Grabow, R. V. Groover, E. R. Laws, Jr., L. R. Elveback, and L. T. Kurland. 1980. Seizures after head trauma: A population study. *Neurology* 30, 683–689.

Annegers, J. F., W. A. Hauser, and L. R. Elveback. 1979a. Remission of seizures and relapse in patients with epilepsy. *Epilepsia* 20, 729–737.

Annegers, J. F., W. A. Hauser, L. R. Elveback, and L. T. Kurland. 1979b. The risk of epilepsy following febrile convulsions. *Neurology* 29, 297–303.

Annegers, J. F., W. A. Hauser, S. B. Shirts, and L. T. Kurland. 1987. Factors prognostic of unprovoked seizures after febrile convulsions. *New England Journal of Medicine* 316, 493–498.

Baird, P. A., and A. D. Sadovnick. 1985. Mental retardation in over half-a-million consecutive livebirths: An epidemiological study. *American Journal of Mental Deficiency* 89, 323–330.

Baldwin, B. T., and L. I. Stecher. 1922. Additional data from consecutive Stanford-Binet Tests. *Journal of Education* 13, 556–560.

Baller, W. R. 1936. A study of the present social status of a group of adults, who, when they were in elementary schools, were classified as mentally deficient. *Genetic Psychology Monographs* 28, 3, 165–244.

Baller, W. R., D. C. Charles, and E. L. Miller. 1967. Mid-life attainment of the mentally retarded: A longitudinal study. *Genetic Psychology Monographs,* 75, 235–329.

Bayley, N. 1970. Development of mental abilities. In *Carmichael's Manual of Child Psychology,* vol. 1, 3rd ed., 1163–1209, ed. P. Mussen. New York: John Wiley & Sons.

———. 1973. *Mental Handicap and Community Care: A Study of Mentally Handicapped People in Sheffield.* London and Boston: Routledge and Kegan Paul.

Benedetti, M. D., S. Shinnar, H. Cohen, D. Inbar, and W. A. Hauser. 1986. Risk factors for epilepsy in children with cerebral palsy and/or mental retardation. *Epilepsia* 27, 614.

Berg, J. M. 1974. Aetiological aspects of mental subnormality: Pathological factors. In A. M. Clarke and A. D. B. Clarke, eds., *Mental deficiency: The changing outlook,* pp. 82–117. London: Methuen.

Berkson, G., and S. Landesman-Dwyer. 1977. Behavioral research on severe and profound mental retardation (1955–1974). *American Journal of Mental Deficiency* 81, 428–454.

Berkson, G. 1983. Repetitive stereotyped behaviors. *American Journal of Mental Deficiency* 88, 239–246.

Bernassi, A., M. Guarino, S. Cammarata, P. Cristoni, M. P. Fantini, A. Ancona, M. Manfredini, and R. D'Alesandro. 1990. An epidemiological study on severe mental retardation among school children in Bologna, Italy. *Developmental Medicine and Child Neurology* 32, 895–901.

Berscheid, E., and E. Walster. 1974. Physical attractiveness. In *Advances in Experimental Social Psychology,* vol. 7, ed. L. Berkowitz. New York: Academic.

Birch, H., S. A. Richardson, Sir D. Baird, G. Horobin, and R. Illsley. 1970. *Mental Subnormality in the Community: A Clinical and Epidemiological Study.* Baltimore: Williams & Wilkins.

Birenbaum, A., and S. Seiffer. 1976. *Resettling retarded adults in a managed community.* New York: Praeger.

Blomquist, H. K.:son, K-H. Gustavson, and G. Holmgren. 1981. Mild mental retardation in children in a northern Swedish county. *Journal of Mental Deficiency Research* 25, 169–186.

Blomquist, H. K.:son, G. Gustavson, G. Holmgren, I. Nordenson, and Palsson-Strae. 1983. Fragile X Syndrome in mildly mentally retarded children in a Northern Swedish county: A prevalence study. *Genetics* 24, 393–398.

British Registrar General's Office. 1951. *Classification of Occupations.* London: HMSO.

Bronfenbrenner, U. 1979. *The Ecology of Human Development.* Cambridge, Mass.: Harvard University Press.

Brown, T. W., E. C. Jenkins, A. C. Gross, C. B. Chan, K. Wisniewski, I. Z. Cohen, and C. M. Miezejeski. 1987. Genetics and expression of the fragile-X syndrome. *Journal of Medical Science* (Uppsala), Supplement 44, 137–154.

Bull, R., and N. Rumsey. 1988. The social psychology of facial disfigurement. In *The Social Psychology of Facial Appearance,* pp. 179–215. New York: Springer-Verlag.

Bunday, S., T. P. Webb, A. Thake, and J. Todd. 1985. A community study of severe mental retardation in the West Midlands and the importance of the fragile-X chromosome in its aetiology. *Journal of Medical Genetics* 22, 258–266.

Bunday, S., A. Thake, and J. Todd. 1989. The recurrence risks for mild idiopathic mental retardation. *Journal of Medical Genetics* 6, 260–266.

Campbell, M., and R. P. Malone. 1991. *Mental Retardation and Psychiatric Disorders* 42, 4, 374–379.

Charles, D. C. 1966. Longitudinal follow-up studies of community adjustment. In *New Vocational Pathways for the Mentally Retarded,* ed. S. De Michael. Washington, D.C.: American Personnel and Guidance Associates.

Clarke, A. M. 1985. Polygenic and environmental interactions. In *Mental Deficiency: The Changing Outlook,* 4th ed., ed. A. M. Clarke, A. D. B. Clarke, and J. M. Berg. London: Methuen.

Clausen, J., ed. 1968. *Socialization and Society.* Boston: Little Brown.

Cobb, H. V. 1972. *The Forecast of Fulfillment: A Review of Research on Predictive Assessment of the Adult Retarded for Social and Vocational Adjustment.* New York and London: Teachers College Press, Columbia University.

Cooper, B., and B. Lackus. 1984. The social-class background of mentally retarded children: A study in Mannheim. *Social Psychiatry* 19, 3–12.

Cooper, B., M. C. Liepmann, K. R. Marker, and P. M. Schieber. 1979. Definition of severe mental retardation in school-age children: Findings of an epidemiological study. *Social Psychiatry* 14, 197–205.

Corbett, J. 1977a. Mental retardation—Psychiatric aspects. In *Child Psychiatry: Modern Approaches,* ed. M. Rutter and L. Hersov, pp. 829–845. London: Blackwell Scientific Publications.

——— 1977b. Population studies of mental retardation. In *Epidemiological Approaches in Child Psychiatry,* ed. P. J. Graham. London: Academic Press.

——— 1979. Psychiatric morbidity and mental retardation. In *Psychiatric Illness and Mental Handicap,* ed. F. E. James and P. P. Snaith, Series B, *British Journal of Psychiatry,* Special Publication.

——— 1981. Epilepsy and mental retardation. In *Epilepsy and Psychiatry,* ed. E. H. Reynolds and M. R. Trimble. Edinburgh: Churchill Livingstone.

——— 1983. An epidemiological approach to the evaluation of services for children with mental retardation. In *Epidemiologic Approaches in Child Psychiatry II,* ed. Schmidt and Remschmidt. New York: Thieme-Stratton.

Corbett, J. A., R. Harris, and R. G. Robinson. 1975. In *Mental Retardation and Developmental Disabilities,* vol. 7, ed. J. Wortis, pp. 79–111. New York: Brunner/Mazel.

Crnic, K. A., W. N. Friedrich, and M. T. Greenberg. 1983. Adaptation of families with mentally retarded children: A model of stress, coping, and family ecology. *American Journal of Mental Deficiency* 88, 125–138.

Czeizel, A., A. Lányi-Engelmayer, L. Klujber, J. Métneki, and G. Tusnády. 1980. Etiological study of mental retardation in Budapest, Hungary. *American Journal of Mental Deficiency* 85, 2, 120–128.

Denckla, M. B., and L. S. James. 1991. An update on autism: A developmental disorder. *Pediatrics,* 87, 5, May Supplement.

Dodd, B., and J. Lechy. 1989. Phonological disorders and mental handicap. In *Language and Communication in Mentally Handicapped People,* ed. M. Beveridge, G. Conti-Ramsden, and J. Luedar. London: Chapman and Hall, p. 36.

Dodrill, C. B., and L. W. Batzel. 1986. Interictal behavioral features of patients with epilepsy. *Epilepsy* 27, Suppl. 2, 64–76.

Drillien, C. M., S. Jameson, and E. M. Wilkinson. 1966. Studies in mental handicap, Part I. Prevalence and distribution by clinical type and severity of defect. *Archives Disease and Child Health* 41, 528–538.

Dugdale, R. 1877. *The Jukes: A Study in Crime, Pauperism, Disease and Heredity.* New York: Putnam.

Edgerton, R. B. 1967, 1993. *The Cloak of Competence.* Berkeley: University of California Press.

Edgerton, R. B., and S. M. Bercovici. 1976. The cloak of competence: years later. *American Journal of Mental Deficiency* 80, 485–497.

Edgerton, R. B., and M. A. Gaston. 1991. *I've Seen It All: Lives of Older Persons with Mental Retardation in the Community.* Baltimore: Paul H. Brookes Publishing.

Einfield, S. L. 1984. Clinical assessment of 4500 developmentally delayed individuals. *Journal of Mental Deficiency Research,* June 28 (part 2), 129–142.

Einfeld, S. L., B. J. Torge, T. Florio, A. Krupinski, M. McLaughlin. 1992. Population prevalence of psychopathology in intellectually handicapped children and adolescents. Abstracts, Ninth World Congress, IASSMD, Broadbeach, Queensland, Australia, Aug. 5–9.

Elwood, J. H., and P. M. Darragh. 1981. Severe mental handicap in Northern Ireland. *Journal of Mental Deficiency Research* 25, 147–155.

Facchini, R. 1995. Self-esteem in young adults with mild mental retardation. Doctoral dissertation, Ferkauf Graduate School of Psychology, Yeshiva University, New York.

Fairbanks, R. 1933. The subnormal child—seventeen years after. *Mental Hygiene* 17, 2, 177–208.

Farber, B. 1968. *Mental Retardation: Its Social Context and Social Consequences.* Boston: Houghton Mifflin.

Farrington, D. P., and D. J. West. 1981. The Cambridge Study in Delinquent Development. In *Prospective Longitudinal Research,* ed. S. A. Mednick and A. E. Baert. Oxford: Oxford University Press.

Ferguson, T., and A. W. Kerr. 1960. *Handicapped Youth.* London: Oxford University Press.

Fleiss, J. L. 1981. *Statistical Methods for Rates and Proportions.* New York: John Wiley & Sons.

Fleiss, J. L., J. Cohen, and B. S. Everitt. 1969. Large sample standard errors of Kappa and weighted Kappa. *Psychological Bulletin* 72, 323–327.

Flynn, J. R. 1987. Massive IQ gains in 14 nations: What IQ tests really measure. *Psychological Bulletin* 101, 2, 171–191.

Folstein, S. E., and J. Piven. 1991. Aetiology of autism: Genetic influences. An update on autism: A developmental disorder. In M. B. Denckla and J. L. Stanley, eds. *Pediatrics* 87, 5, May Suppl.

Forsyth, J. P., J. D. Nisbet, and J. McKinnon. 1976. *Provision for Special Education in Aberdeen, 1945–1975: A Base Study in Educational Development.* Aberdeen: Department of Education, University of Aberdeen. February.

Frost, J. B. 1984. Behavioral disturbance in mentally handicapped adults. In *Perspectives and Progress in Mental Retardation,* vol. 2, *Biomedical Aspects,* ed. J. M. Berg, pp. 299–308. Baltimore: University Park Press.

Fryers, T. 1984. *The Epidemiology of Severe Intellectual Impairment.* London: Academic Press.

——— 1987. Epidemiological issues in mental retardation. *Journal of Mental Deficiency Research* 31, 365–384.

——— 1990, 1991. Mental retardation and epidemiology. *Current Opinion in Psychiatry* 3, 595–602; 4, 662–666.

——— 1992. Epidemiology and taxonomy in mental retardation. *Paediatric and Perinatal Epidemiology* 6, 181–192.

Gallagher, J. J. 1985. The prevalence of mental retardation: Cross-cultural considerations from Sweden and the United States. *Intelligence* 9, 97–108.

Garber, H. 1988. *The Milwaukee Project.* Washington, D.C.: American Association on Mental Retardation.

Gillberg, C. 1984. Infantile autism and other childhood psychoses in a Swedish urban region: Epidemiological aspects. *Journal of Child Psychiatry,* January 25 (1), 35–43.

Gillberg, C., M. Persson, M. Grafman, and U. Themner. 1986. Psychiatric disorders in mildly and severely mentally retarded urban children and adolescents: Epidemiological aspects. *British Journal of Psychiatry* 149, 68–74.

Gillberg, C., B. Svenson, G. Carlstrom, E. Waldenstrom, and P. Rasmussen. 1983. Mental retardation in Swedish urban children: Some epidemiological considerations. *Applied Research in Mental Retardation* 4, 207–218.

Goddard, H. 1912. *The Kallikak Family: A Study in the Heredity of Feeblemindedness.* New York: Macmillan.

Goffman, E. 1963. *Stigma: Notes on the Management of Spoiled Identity.* Englewood Cliffs, N.J.: Prentice-Hall.

Gold, M. W. 1972. Research on the vocational habilitation of the retarded: The present, the future. In *International Review of Research in Mental Retardation,* vol. 6, ed. N. R. Ellis. New York: Academic Press.

Goldstein, H. 1964. Social and occupational adjustment. In *Mental Retardation,* ed. H. A. Stevens and R. Heber. Chicago and London: University of Chicago Press.

Gordon, N. 1991. Specific disorders of learning: Motor skills, language, and behavior. In *Paediatric Neurology,* ed. E. M. Brett. Edinburgh: Churchill Livingstone.

Gostason, R. 1985. Psychiatric illness among the mentally retarded—A Swedish population study. *Acta Psychiatrica Scandinavica,* suppl. 318.

Gould, J. 1976. Language development and non-verbal skills in severely mentally retarded children: An epidemiological study. *Journal of Mental Deficiency Research* 20, 129.

Goulden, K. J., and S. Shinnar. 1989. Is epilepsy a risk factor for behavior disturbance in children with multiple developmental disabilities? Presented in part at annual meeting of the Child Neurology Society, Halifax, Nova Scotia.

Goulden, K. J., S. Shinnar, H. Koller, M. Katz, and S. A. Richardson. 1992. Epilepsy in children with mental retardation: A cohort study. *Epilepsia* 32, 5, 690–697.

Gower, W. 1881. *Epilepsy and Other Chronic Convulsive Disorders.* London: Churchill.

Granat, K., and S. Granat. 1973. Below average intelligence and mental retardation. *American Journal of Mental Deficiency* 78, 1, 27–31.

Gruenberg, E. M. 1955. A special census of suspected referred mental retardation, Onondaga County, New York. Pp. 84–127 in *Technical Report of the Mental Health Research Unit.* New York State Dept. of Mental Hygiene. Syracuse: Syracuse University Press.

Gruenberg, E. M. 1964. Epidemiology. In *Mental Retardation: A Review of Research,* ed. H. A. Stevens and R. Heber, pp. 259–306. Chicago: University of Chicago Press.

Gunzberg, H. C. 1974. Psychotherapy. In *Mental Deficiency. The Changing Outlook,* 3rd ed., ed. A. M. Clarke and A. D. B. Clarke. London: Methuen.

Gustavson, K.-H., G. Holmgren, and H. K.:son Blomquist. 1987. Chromosomal aberrations in mildly mentally retarded children in a Northern Swedish county. *Uppsala Journal of Medical Science,* suppl. 44, 165–168.

Gustavson, K-H., G. Holmgren, R. Jonsell, and H. K.:son Blomquist. 1977a. Severe mental retardation in children in a northern Swedish county. *Journal of Mental Deficiency Research* 21, 161.

Gustavson, K-H., B. Hagberg, G. Hagberg, K. Sars. 1977b. Severe mental retardation in a Swedish county. I. Epidemiology, gestational age, birthweight, and associated CNS handicaps in children born 1959–70. *Acta Paediatrica Scandinavica* 66, 373–379.

—— 1977c. Severe mental retardation in a Swedish county. II. Etiologic and pathogenetic aspects of children born 1959–70. *Neuropaediatrie* 8, 293–304.

Grossman, H. J., ed. 1983. *Classification in Mental Retardation.* Washington, D.C.: American Association on Mental Deficiency.

Haan, N. 1963. Proposed model of ego functioning: Coping and defense mechanisms in relationship to IQ change. *Psychology Monographs* 77, 8.

Hagberg, B., G. Hagberg, A. Lewerth, and U. Lindberg. 1981a. Mild mental retardation in Swedish school children. I. Prevalence. *Acta Paediatrica Scandinavica* 70, 441–444.

—— 1981b. Mild mental retardation in Swedish school children. II. Etiologic and pathogenic aspects. *Acta Paediatrica Scandinavica* 70, 445–452.

Hagberg, B., and M. Kylleman. 1983. Epidemiology of mental retardation—A Swedish survey. *Brain and Development* 5, 5, 441–449.

Harter, S. 1982. The perceived competency scale for children. *Child Development* 53, 87–97.

Hauser, W. A., and L. T. Kurland. 1975. The epidemiology of epilepsy in Rochester, Minnesota, 1935 through 1967. *Epilepsia* 16, 1–66.

Hauser, W. A., S. Shinnar, H. Cohen, D. Inbar, and M. D. Benedetti. 1987. Clinical predictors of epilepsy among children with cerebral palsy and/or mental retardation. *Neurology* 37, suppl. 1, 150.

Homans, G. C. 1950. *The Human Group.* New York: Harcourt, Brace.

—— 1961. *Social Behavior: Its Elementary Forms.* New York: Harcourt, Brace.

Honzik, M. P., J. W. McFarlane, and L. Allen. 1948. The stability of mental test performance between two and eighteen years. *Journal of Experimental Education* 17, 309–324.

Iivanainen, M. 1981. Neurological examination of the mentally retarded child: Evidence of central nervous system abnormality. In *Assessing the Handicaps and Needs of Mentally Retarded Children,* ed. B. Cooper. London: Academic Press.

Innes, G., A. W. Johnston, and W. M. Millar. 1978. *Mental Subnormality in North East Scotland: A Multi-Disciplinary Study of Total Population.* Scottish Health Services Studies no. 38, Scottish Home and Health Department.

Israel, H. 1980. The fundamentals of cranial and facial growth. In *Human growth,* ed. J. M. Tanner and F. Faulkner. New York: Plenum.

Jackson, R. 1977. Post-school adjustment of the mentally retarded: A critical note on the Nebraskan Longitudinal Survey of Baller, Charles, and Miller. *Journal Mental Deficiency Research* 21, 273.

Jensen, A. R. 1981. Raising the IQ: The Ramey and Haskis study. *Intelligence* 5, 29–40.

Kaariainen, R., P. Piepponen, and T. Vaskilampi, eds. 1985. *A Multidisciplinary Case-Control Study of Mental Retardation in Children ofFour Birth Cohorts.* Publications of the University of Kuopio.

Kagan, J. 1964. Acquisition and significance of sex typing and sex role identity. In *Review of Child Development Research,* ed. M. L. Hoffman and L. W. Hoffman. New York: Russell Sage Foundation.

Kanner, L. A. 1964. *A History of the Care and Study of the Mentally Retarded.* Springfield, Ill.: Charles C. Thomas.

Kaplan, E. L., and P. Meier. 1958. Nonparametric estimation for incomplete observations. *Journal of the American Statistical Association* 53, 457–481.

Kennedy, R. J. 1948. *The Social Adjustment of Morons in a Connecticut City.* Report of the Commission to Survey the Human Resources of Connecticut. Hartford, Conn.: Mansfield-Southbury Training Schools.

——— 1966. *A Connecticut Community Revisited: A Study of the Social Adjustment of a Group of Mentally Deficient Adults in 1948 and 1960.* Hartford, Conn.: Connecticut State Department of Health, Office of Mental Retardation.

Kevles, D. J. 1984. Annals of eugenics: A secular faith. In four parts in *The New Yorker:* Oct. 8, pp. 51–115; Oct. 15, pp. 52–125; Oct. 22, pp. 92–150; Oct. 29, pp. 51–114.

Kiely, M. 1987. The prevalence of mental retardation. *Epidemiological Reviews* 9, 194–218.

Koegel, P., and R. B. Edgerton. 1984. Black "six-hour retarded children" as young adults. In *Lives in Process: Mildly Retarded Adults in a Large City,* ed. R. B. Edgerton. Monographs of the American Association of Mental Deficiency, no. 6. C. E. Meyer, series ed. Washington, D.C.: American Association on Mental Deficiency.

Koller, H., S. A. Richardson, and M. Katz. 1984. Estimating the prevalence of mild mental retardation in the adult years. *Journal of Mental Deficiency Research* 28, 101–107.

——— 1988a. Peer relationships of mildly retarded young adults living in the community. *Journal of Mental Deficiency Research* 32, 321–331.

——— 1988b. Marriage in a young adult mentally retarded population. *Journal of Mental Deficiency Research* 32, 93–102.

——— 1992. Families of children with mental retardation: Comprehensive view from an epidemiologic perspective. *American Journal on Mental Retardation* 97, 3, 315–332.

Koller, H., S. A. Richardson, M. Katz, and J. McLaren. 1982. Behavior disturbance in childhood and the early adult years in populations who were and were not mentally retarded. *Journal of Preventive Psychiatry* 1, 4, 453–467.

——— 1983. Behavior disturbance since childhood among a 5-year birth cohort of all mentally retarded young adults in a city. *American Journal of Mental Deficiency* 87, 4, 386–395.

Kushlick, A., and R. Blunden. 1974. The epidemiology of mental subnormality. In *Mental Deficiency: The Changing Outlook,* 3rd ed., ed. A. M. Clarke and A. D. B. Clarke, pp. 31–81. London: Methuen.

Lagergren, J. 1981. Children with motor handicaps: Epidemiological, medical, and socio-paediatric aspects of motor-handicapped children in a Swedish county. *Acta Paediatrica Scandinavica* 70, suppl. 289, 1–71.

Lamont, M. A., and N. R. Dennis. 1988. Aetiology of mild mental retardation. *Archives of Disease in Children* 63, 1032–1038.

Lamont, M. A., N. R. Dennis, and M. Seabright. 1986. Chromosome abnormalities in pupils attending ESN/M schools. *Archives of Diseases in Childhood* 61, 223–226.

Lapouse, R., and M. Weitzner. 1970. Epidemiology. In *Mental Retardation: An Annual Review,* ed. J. Wortis. New York: Grune and Stratton.

Lemkau, P. V., and P. D. Imre. 1968. Results of a field epidemiological study. *American Journal of Mental Deficiency* 73, 858–863.

Levinson, E. J. 1962. *Children in Maine.* Orono: University of Maine Press.

Littler, C. R., and G. Salomon. 1985. The design of jobs. In *The Experience of Work,* ed. C. R. Littler. Hampshire, England: Gower Publishing, pp. 85–104.

Lubchenko, L., C. Hansman, and E. Boyd. 1966. Intrauterine growth in length and head circumference as estimated from live birth at gestational ages from 26 to 42 weeks. *Pediatrics* 37, 403.

MacEachron, A. E. 1979. Mentally retarded offenders: Prevalence and characteristics. *American Journal of Mental Deficiency* 84, 165–176.

Martindale, A., E. McGrath, G. P. Hosking, and R. A. Buckley. 1988. Trends in the prevalence of severe mental handicap in Sheffield since 1960. *Community Medicine* 10, 4, 331–340.

May, D. R. 1981. The Aberdeen Delinquency Study. In *Prospective Longitudinal Research,* ed. S. A. Mednick and A. E. Baert. Oxford: Oxford University Press.

McDonald, A. D. 1973. Severely retarded children in Quebec: Prevalence, causes, and care. *American Journal of Mental Deficiency* 78, 2, 205–215.

McLaren, J. 1988. Kathleen. In *Living with Mental Handicap: Transition in the Lives of People with Mental Handicap.* Research Highlight in Social Work, 16, ed. G. Horobin and D. May. London: Jessica Kingsley Publishers.

McLaren, J., and S. E. Bryson. 1987. Review of recent epidemiological studies of mental retardation: Prevalence, associated disorders, and etiology. *American Journal on Mental Retardation* 92, 3, 243–54.

McQueen, P. C., M. W. Spence, B. J. Garner, L. H. Pereira, and E. J. J. Windsor. 1987. Prevalence of major mental retardation and associated disabilities in the Canadian Maritime Provinces. *American Journal of Mental Deficiency* 91, 5, 460–466.

Mellsop, G. W. 1974. Psychiatric patients seen as children and adults: Childhood predictors of adult illness. In *Annual Progress in Child Psychiatry and Child Development,* ed. S. Chess and A. Thomas. New York: Brunner/Mazel.

Mercer, J. R. 1966. Patterns of family crisis related to reacceptance of the retarded. *American Journal of Mental Deficiency* 71, 19–32.

Miller, E. L. 1965. Ability and social adjustment at midlife of persons earlier judged mentally deficient. *Genetic Psychology Monographs* 72, 139–198.

Mittleman, M., Z. Stein, M. Susser, and L. Belmont. 1978. Psychiatric sickness and cognitive function: A causal connection? In *Cognitive Defects in the Development of Mental Illness,* ed. G. S. Serban. New York: Brunner/Mazel.

Mittler, P. 1974. Language and communication. In *Mental Deficiency,* 3rd ed., ed. A. M. Clarke and A. D. B. Clarke. London: Methuen.

——— 1979. *People Not Patients.* London: Methuen.

Moriarty, A. E. 1966. *Constancy and IQ Change: A Clinical View of Relationships between Tested Intelligence and Personality.* Springfield, Ill.: Charles C. Thomas.

Munro, J. D. 1986. Epidemiology and the extent of mental retardation. *Psychiatric Clinics of North America* 9, 4, 591–624.

Murphy, C. C., M. Yeargin-Allsop, P. Decoufle, and C. D. Drews. 1995. The administrative prevalence of mental retardation in 10-year-old children in metropolitan Atlanta, 1985 through 1987. *American Journal of Public Health* 85, 3, 319–328.

Nellhaus, G. 1968. Head circumference from birth to eighteen years: Practical composite international and interracial graphs. *Pediatrics* 41, 106.

Nelson, K. B., and J. H. Ellenberg. 1976. Predictors of epilepsy in children who have experienced febrile seizures. *New England Journal of Medicine* 295, 1029–1033.

Nihira, K., R. Foster, M. Shellhaas, and H. Leland. 1974. *Adaptive Behavior Scale.* Washington, D.C.: American Association on Mental Deficiency.

Nihira, K., C. E. Meyers, and I. T. Mink. 1980. Home environment, family adjustment, and the development of mentally retarded children. *Applied Research in Mental Retardation* 1, 5–24.

Ounsted, C., J. Lindsay, and P. Richards. 1987. Temporal lobe epilepsy, 1948–1986: A biographical study. *Clinics in Developmental Medicine,* 103, McKeith Press. Philadelphia: J. B. Lippincott.

Penrose, L. S. 1949. *The Biology of Mental Defect.* London: Sigwick and Jackson, p. 45.

Peto, R., and J. Peto. 1972. Asymptotically efficient rank invariant test procedures. *Journal of Research of the Statistical Society(A)* 135, 185–206.

Ramer, T. 1946. *The Prognosis of Mentally Retarded Children.* State Institute of Human Genetics and Race Biology. Uppsala, Boktrycheri: A. B. Bennel.

——— 1946. The prognosis of mentally retarded children. *Acta Psychiatrica Neurological Supplement* 41, 1–142.

Rantakallio, P., and L. von Wendt. 1986. Mental retardation and subnormality in a birth cohort of 12,000 children in Northern Finland. *American Journal Mental Deficiency* 90, 380–387.

Reid, A. H. 1985. Psychiatric disorders. In *Mental Deficiency: The Changing Outlook,* 4th ed., ed. A. M. Clarke, A. D. Clarke, and J. M. Berg. London: Methuen.

Reiter, S., and A. M. Levi. 1980. Factors affecting social integration of noninstitutionalized mentally retarded adults. *American Journal of Mental Deficiency* 85, 25–30.

Richardson, S. A. 1968. The effect of physical disability on the socialization of a child. In *The Handbook of Socialization, Theory, and Research,* ed. D. A. Goslin, pp. 1047–1064. New York: Rand McNally.

——— 1976. Attitudes and behavior toward the physically handicapped. In Developmental disabilities: Psychologic and social implications, ed. D. Bergsma and A. E. Pulver. *National Foundation, March of Dimes, Birth Defects,* Original Article Series, III(4), 15–34.

——— 1983. Children's values in regard to disabilities: A reply to Yuker. *Rehabilitation Psychology* 28, 3, 14–23.

——— 1984. Deinstitutionalization and institutionalization of children with mental retardation. In A. E. Siegel and H. W. Stevenson, eds., *Child Development and Social Policy* 1, 318–366. Chicago: University of Chicago Press.

Richardson, S. A., B. S. Dohrenwend, and D. Klein. 1965. *Interviewing: Its Forms and Functions.* New York: Basic Books.

Richardson, S. A., K. J. Goulden, H. Koller, and M. Katz. 1990. The long-term influence of the family of upbringing on young adults with mild mental retardation. In *Key Issues in Mental Retardation Research,* ed. W. Fraser, pp. 190–202. London: Routledge.

Richardson, S. A., M. Katz, and H. Koller. 1993. Patterns of leisure activities of young adults with mild mental retardation. *American Journal on Mental Retardation,* 97, 4, 431–442.

——— 1994. Leisure activities of young adults not receiving mental handicap services who were in a special school for mental handicap as children. *Journal of Intellectual Disability Research* 38, 163–175.

Richardson, S. A., and H. Koller. 1985. Epidemiology. In *Mental Deficiency: The Changing Outlook,* 4th ed., ed. A. M. Clarke, A. D. B. Clarke, and J. Berg. London: Methuen.

——— 1992. Vulnerability and resilience in adults who were classified as mildly mentally handicapped in childhood. In *Vulnerability and Resilience in Human Development,* ed. B. Tizard and V. Varma. London: Jessica Kingsley Publishers.

——— 1994. The epidemiology of mental retardation. In *The Epidemiology of Childhood Disorders,* ed. B. Pless. London: Oxford University Press.

Richardson, S. A., H. Koller, and M. Katz. 1985a. Relationship of upbringing to later behavior disturbance of mildly mentally retarded young people. *American Journal of Mental Deficiency* 9, 1, 1–8.

——— 1985b. Continuities and change in behavior disturbance: A follow-up study of mildly retarded young people. *American Journal of Orthopsychiatry* 55, 2 (April), 220–229.

——— 1985c. Appearance and mental retardation: Some first steps in the development and application of a measure. *American Journal of Mental Deficiency* 89, 5, 475–484.

Richardson, S. A., H. Koller, and M. Katz. 1986a. Factors leading to differences in the school performance of boys and girls. *Developmental and Behavioral Pediatrics* 7, 1.

Richardson, S. A., M. Katz, and H. Koller. 1986b. Sex differences in number of children administratively classified as mildly mentally retarded: An epidemiological review. *American Journal of Mental Deficiency* 91, 3, 250–256.

Richardson, S. A., H. Koller, and M. Katz. 1988. Job histories in open employment of a population of young adults with mental retardation: I. *American Journal on Mental Retardation* 9, 2, 483–491.

Richardson, S. A., H. Koller, M. Katz, and J. McLaren. 1981. A functional classification of seizures and its distribution in a mentally retarded population. *American Journal of Mental Deficiency* 85, 475–486.

——— 1984a. Career paths through mental retardation services: An epidemiological perspective. *Applied Research in Mental Retardation* 5, 53–67.

—— 1984b. Patterns of disability in a mentally retarded population between ages 16 and 22 years. In *Perspectives and Progress in Mental Retardation,* vol. 2, *Biomedical Aspects,* ed. J. M. Berg, pp. 25–37. Baltimore: University Park Press.

Rosenbrock, H. 1985. Eugenics and the work that people do. In *The Experience of Work,* ed. C. P. Littler, p. 161–171. Hampshire: Gower Publishing.

Ross, R. T., M. J. Begab, E. H. Dondes, J. S. Gianpiccolo, and C. E. Meyers. 1985. *Lives of the Mentally Retarded: A Forty-year Follow-up Study.* Stanford: Stanford University Press.

Rutter, M. 1973. Relationships between child and adult psychiatric disorders. In *Annual Progress in Child Psychiatry and Child Development,* ed. S. Chess and A. Thomas. New York: Brunner/Mazel.

Rutter, M., P. Graham, and W. Yule. 1970. *A Neuropsychiatric Study in Childhood.* London: Spastics International Medical Publications in assoc. with Wm. Heinemann Medical Books.

Rutter, M., and N. Madge. 1981. *Cycles of disadvantage.* London: Heinemann.

Rutter, M., D. Shaffer, and M. Shepherd. 1975. *A Multiaxial Classification of Child Psychiatric Disorders.* Geneva: World Health Organization.

Rutter, M., J. Tizard, and K. Whitmore. 1970. *Education, Health, and Behavior.* London: Longman Group (reprint, 1981, Huntington, New York: Krieger).

Rutter, M., J. Tizard, W. Yule, P. Graham, and K. Whitmore. 1977. Isle of Wight Studies, 1964–1974. In *Annual Progress in Child Psychiatry and Child Development,* ed. S. Chess and A. Thomas. New York: Brunner/Mazel.

Saenger, G. 1957. *The Adjustment of Severely Retarded Adults in the Community.* A Report to the New York State Interdepartmental Health Resources Board. Albany, N.Y., October.

Salazar, A. M., B. Jabbari, S. C. Vance, J. Grafman, D. Amin, and J. D. Dillon. 1985. Epilepsy after penetrating head injury. I, Clinical correlates. *Neurology* 35, 1406–1414.

Santamour, M. B., and B. West. 1979. The mentally retarded offender in the social context. *Amicus,* Jan./Feb.

Scheerenberger, R. C. 1983. *A History of Mental Retardation.* Baltimore: Brookes Publishing.

Shaffer, D. 1977. Brain damage and psychiatric illness. In M. Rutter and L. Hersov, eds., *Child psychiatry: Modern approaches,* pp. 185–215. London: Blackwell Scientific Publications.

Shepherd, C., and G. Hosking. 1989. Epilepsy in school children with intellectual impairment in Sheffield: The size and nature of the problem and the implications for service provision. *Journal of Mental Deficiency Research* 33, 511–514.

Shiotsuki, Y., T. Matsuishi, K. Yoshimura, F. Yamashita, K. Yano, H. Tokimasa,

and H. Shoji. 1984. The prevalence of mental retardation (MR) in Kurume City. *Brain Development* 6, 487–490.
Skeels, H. M. 1966. Adult status of children with contrasting early life experience. *Monographs of the Society for Research in Child Development* 31 (3 serial, no. 105.)
Skeels, H. M., and H. B. Dye. 1939. The study of the effects of differential stimulation on mentally retarded children. *Proceedings and Addresses of the American Association of Mental Deficiency* 44, 114–136.
Skeels, H. M., R. Updegraff, B. L. Wellman, and H. M. Williams. 1938. A study of environmental stimulation: an orphanage preschool project. *University of Iowa Studies in Child Welfare* 15, 4.
Sonnander, K. 1990. Prevalence of mental retardation: An empirical study of an unselected school population. In *Key Issues in Mental Retardation Research,* ed. W. I. Fraser. London: Routledge.
Sorel, F. 1974. *The Prevalence of Mental Retardation.* The Netherlands: Tellberg University Press.
Stein, Z., and M. Susser. 1960. The families of dull children: A classification for predicting careers. *British Journal of Preventive Social Medicine* 14, 83–88.
——— 1963. The social distribution of mental retardation. *American Journal of Mental Deficiency,* 67, 811–821.
Stein, Z., M. Susser, and G. Saenger. 1976. Mental retardation in a national population of young men in the Netherlands. II, Prevalence of mild mental retardation. *American Journal of Epidemiology* 104, 2, 159–169.
Stein, Z., M. Susser, G. Saenger, and F. Marolla. 1975. *Famine and Human Development: The Dutch Hunger Winter of 1944–1945.* New York: Oxford University Press.
Sugiyama, T., Y. Takei, and A. Tokuichiro. 1992. Neurobiology of infantile autism. In *The Proceedings of the International Symposium on Neurobiology of Infantile Autism,* Tokyo, 10–11 Nov. 1990. Ed. H. Naruse and E. M. Ornitz. Amsterdam: Excerpta-Medica.
Susser, M., W. A. Hauser, J. L. Kiely, N. Paneth, and Z. Stein. 1985. Quantitative estimates of prenatal and perinatal risk factors for perinatal mortality, cerebral palsy, mental retardation, and epilepsy. In *Prenatal and perinatal factors associated with brain disorders,* ed. J. M. Freeman. Bethesda, Maryland: National Institutes of Health; NIH publication no. 85–1149, 359–440.
Tarjan, G. 1970. Some thoughts on social-cultural retardation. In *Socio-cultural Aspects of Mental Retardation,* ed. H. C. Haywood, pp. 745–758. New York: Appleton-Century-Crofts.
——— 1977. Mental retardation and clinical psychiatry. In *Research to Practice in Mental Retardation,* ed. P. Mittler, 1, 401–407. Baltimore: University Park Press.

Terman, L., and M. Merrill. 1973. Stanford Binet Intelligence Scale: Manual for the third revision. Form L-N. Boston: Houghton Mifflin.

Thake, A., J. Todd, T. Webb, and S. Bunday. 1987. Children with the Fragile-X chromosome at schools for the mildly mentally retarded. *Developmental Medicine and Child Neurology* 29, 711–719.

Tizard, J. 1964. *Community Services for the Mentally Handicapped.* London: Oxford University Press.

——— 1965. Longitudinal and follow-up studies. In *Mental Deficiency: The Changing Outlook,* 2nd ed., ed. A. M. Clarke and A. D. B. Clarke. London: Methuen.

Tredgold, A. F. 1908. *Mental Deficiency.* London: Balliere, Tindall & Cox.

Turnbull, A. P., J. A. Summers, and M. J. Brotherson. 1986. Family life cycle. In *Families of Handicapped Persons,* ed. J. J. Gallagher and P. M. Vietze, pp. 45–66. Baltimore: Brookes.

Turner, A., A. Daniel, and M. Frost. 1980. Heterozygous expression of X-linked mental retardation and X Chromosome marker: Fragile (X) (q27). *New England Journal of Medicine* 303, 662–664.

Turner, J. L. 1983. Workshop society: Ethnographic observations in a work setting for retarded adults. In *Environments and Behavior: The Adaptation of Mentally Retarded Persons,* ed. K. T. Kernan, M. J. Begab, and R. B. Edgerton, pp. 147–171. Baltimore: University Park Press.

von Wendt, L., P. Rantakallio, A.-L. Saukkonen, and H. Makinen. 1985. Epilepsy and associated handicaps in a one-year birth cohort in Northern Finland. *European Journal of Pediatrics* 144, 149–151.

Wald, I., E. Zdzienicka, M. Bartnik, A. Kalinska, and K. Mrugalska. 1977. *The Ten Years Follow-up Study of a Representative Sample of the Low-grade Mentally Retarded in Poland.* Warsaw: Psychoneurological Institute.

Wallner, T. 1988. The number of mentally retarded—A result of steps taken by society? Changes in the age structure among mentally retarded persons in Sweden, 1973–1982. *Developmental Disabilities* 9, 135–143.

Werner, E. E., and R. S. Smith. 1980. An epidemiologic perspective on some antecedents and consequences of childhood mental health problems and learning disabilities. In *Annual progress in child psychiatry and child development,* ed. S. Chess and A. Thomas, pp. 133–147. New York: Brunner/Mazel.

Whitman, S., and B. B. Hermann. 1986. *Psychopathology in Epilepsy: Social Dimensions.* New York: Oxford University Press.

Windle, C. D. 1962. Prognosis of Mental Subnormals, *Monograph Supplement, American Journal of Mental Deficiency* 66, 1–180.

Wohlwill, J. F. 1980. Cognitive development in childhood. In *Constancy and Change in Human Development,* ed. O. G. Brim, Jr., and J. Kagan, pp. 359–444. Cambridge, Mass.: Harvard University Press.

World Health Organization. 1980. *International Classification of Impairments, Disabilities, and Handicaps.* Geneva: World Health Organization.

——— 1985. *Mental Retardation: Meeting the Challenge.* WHO Offset publication no. 86. Geneva: WHO.

Wright, B. 1983. Physical disability. In *Physical Disability: A Psychosocial Approach,* 2nd ed. New York: Harper and Row.

Zigler, E. 1995. Editorial: Can we "cure" mild mental retardation among individuals in the lower socioeconomic stratum? *American Journal of Public Health* 85, 3, 302–304.

Index

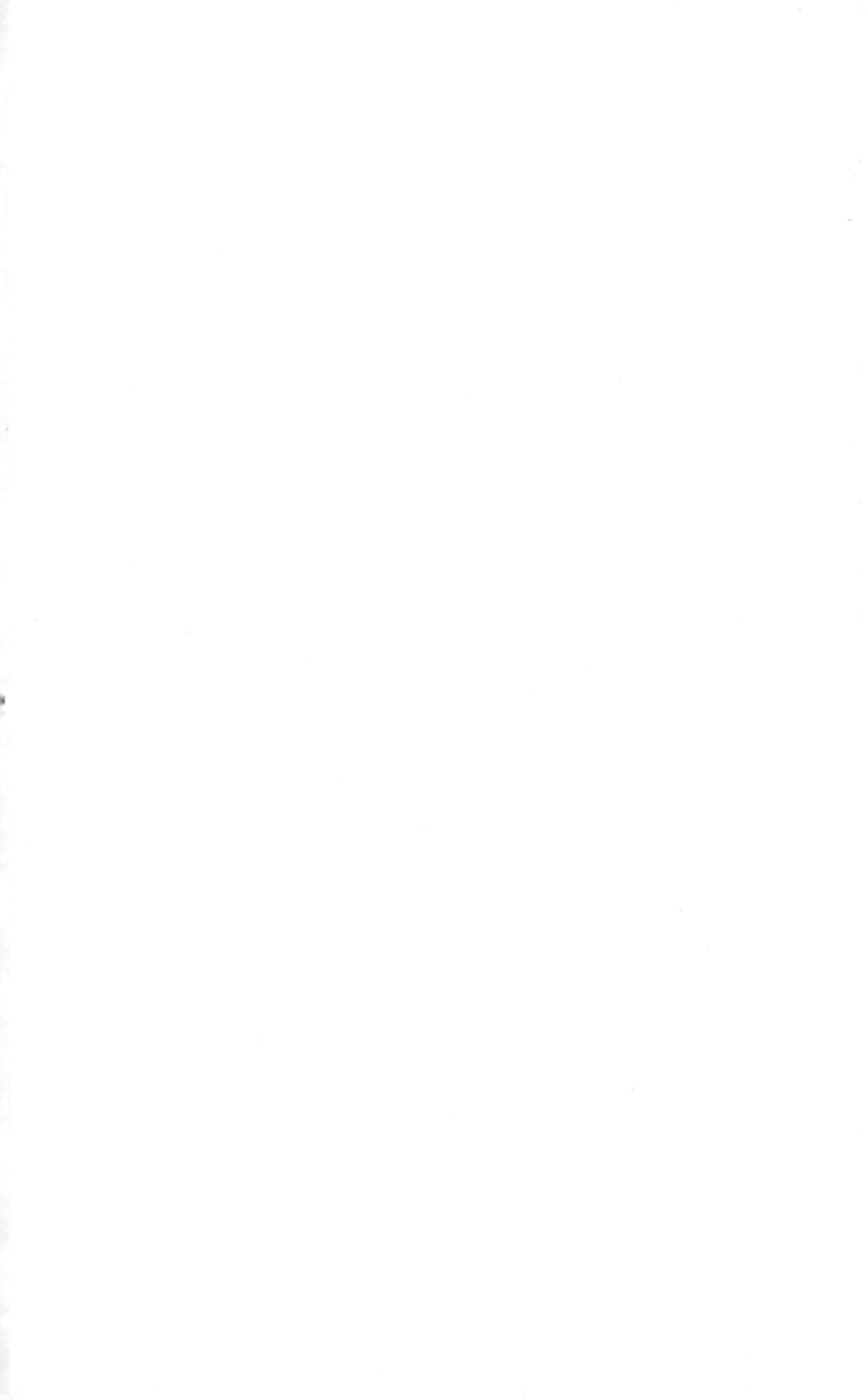

NORTHERN MICHIGAN UNIVERSITY
3 1854 005 709 434